The Sirtfood Diet

A Beginner's Guide to Losing Weight, Burning Fat, Getting Lean, and Staying Healthy With Carnivore, Vegetarian, and Vegan Recipes to Activate Your Skinny Gene

Adele T. Cook

contained within this document, including, but not limited to, errors, omissions, or inaccuracies.

Table of Contents

Introduction

Do you want to lose weight without compromising your health? Are you sick and tired of fad diets that starve your body and drain your wallet? Do you want a clear, simple, affordable, and sustainable diet plan you can follow on any budget, and on the busiest schedule? If so, *The Sirtfood Diet: A Beginner's Guide to Losing Weight, Burning Fat, Getting Lean, and Staying Healthy With Carnivore, Vegetarian, and Vegan Recipes to Activate Your Skinny Gene* is the right book for you! This book will show you how, when, what, and how much to eat.

In theory, slimming down is a simple process. Eat fewer calories than you burn, right? Except that, unless you find a way to craft a healthy, abundant diet, your metabolism will slow down. You won't lose weight long-term despite having reduced calorie intake. Have you ever wondered why this happens?

The answer is that most fad diets eventually boil down to a repetitive pattern of eating a limited number of nutrient-poor foods. A successful diet plan is both delicious and healthy, not just low on calories. The reason why this is so important is that there are many important, but less heard of nutrients your diet needs to include. Vitamins, minerals, and fiber are only at the tip of the iceberg of nutrients and biochemicals that are vital for weight loss. The latest research shows that sirtuin proteins, whose levels increase with the intake of 20 superfoods this diet is based on, help you not only burn fat but also improve your long-term health. That's right! And the best part is that your diet doesn't have to be completely limited to these 20 foods! The Sirtfood diet includes and emphasizes these foods as an addition to an otherwise healthy, clean diet to boost your weight loss.

The Sirtfood diet became popular after many celebrities who've struggled with weight, like Adele and Pippa Middleton used it to shed pounds and achieve a healthy weight without compromising health.

In this book, you will first learn the basics of the Sirtfood diet. To apply this simple principle into your daily routine and design a sustainable meal plan, you'll need to know what the so-called "Sirtfoods" do to your body, and how they lead to weight loss. This will help you not only understand the importance of these foods, but also make connections between how your diet looks like now, and what you need to change to transition into your new diet plan more easily. For starters, you will learn the basic premise and the science behind the Sirtfood diet. You will learn what exactly the sirtuin proteins are, what they do, and how the foods you eat affect their levels in your body.

In this book, you will also learn about the newly discovered "skinny gene," and how it relates to the Sirtfood diet. That's right! The latest research confirmed the existence of this gene in animals and humans, and this book will give you the basic instructions for how to unlock your hidden potentials to lose weight. You will learn how to activate this gene throughout a three-phase process of the Sirtfood diet plan and implement its principles into your eating habits for the rest of your life to maintain health and weight loss. Eating habits are the second most important weight loss factor that can make or break your efforts to achieve the desired weight. In this book, we'll delve into how the three main phases of the Sirtfood diet change your metabolism, and how you need to proceed so that your progress remains permanent.

Once you've learned the basics of the Sirtfood Diet, you'll move on to learn how to use it to burn fat and build up muscle mass. One of the biggest flaws of common fad diets is that they lead to short-term loss of water, and then muscle loss, instead of fat burning. This happens because most common diets restrict the intake of protein and carb-rich foods. As a result, your body doesn't get enough of the basic substances it needs to build muscle tissue, and it starts burning your muscle tissue instead of fat to compensate for the lack of energy. In this book, you will learn how and why the Sirtfood diet helps maintain your muscle mass, and even build it up if you want a more robust physique.

After you've learned the basics of the Sirtfood diet and its application, you will discover everything about the 20 Sirt Foods that spark sirtuin proteins and the activation of the so-called "skinny gene." Simply listing these foods won't be enough to put you on the right track. You'll need to know why and how these specific foods help you lose weight and boost health and the amounts needed to consume so that you reap their nutritional benefits. More importantly, you'll learn many creative ideas for how to prepare these foods to preserve their nutrients and enhance the flavor.

After understanding which foods to include in your diet for speedy long-term weight loss, you will learn how to make simple, fast, and delicious Sirtfood meals across different stages of this diet. This is the part where the fun begins!

The second half of this book will give you easy and delicious recipes you can cook on any budget, regardless of how busy you are. This book will show you how to Sirtify your diet from breakfast to dinner, whether you're following a carnivore, vegetarian, vegan, or keto diet. That's right! You can enrich your diet with sirtuin-boosting foods even if you're currently following a different diet plan! All that with highly specific recipes with a calorie and nutrient value breakdown, shopping lists, and a step-by-step cooking guide.

Now, sit back and enjoy it! As you dig into this book, rest assured that all you need to do is learn and apply the tips, suggestions, and recipes, and watch your body slim down. More importantly, you will boost your health and immune system, and prevent many diet-related illnesses from developing. Good luck on your journey!

Chapter 1:

What Is the Sirtfood diet?

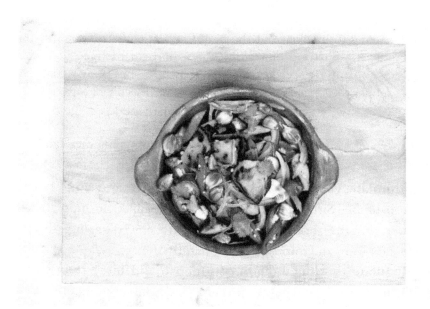

Despite the diet's popularity across the globe, many people still don't understand what the Sirtfood diet is all about. Perhaps, you like the idea of being able to enjoy wine and chocolate while losing weight. Or, you smile at the prospect of losing weight just by adding a couple of "magic" foods to your meals. While all of this is accurate and possible, it's still necessary for you to get the full scope of how the Sirtfood concept affects your body, and how to use it to reap the maximum health benefits. Your journey here will start with an introduction to the Sirtfood diet. In this chapter, you'll find out about the diet's main principles, effects on the body, and how it works. This will help you set reasonable expectations and understand how to design your meals.

The Science Behind Sirtfood Diet

Despite what some people think, the Sirtfood diet isn't just another seasonal fad or hype doomed to disappear. On the contrary. As this concept can be integrated into a multitude of lifestyles and diet plans, it is likely to stay as one of the memorable postulates for boosting one's metabolism and health. The same way even those who don't follow the Keto diet became more aware of the benefits that come from reducing carbohydrates, the Sirtfood diet can leave a permanent trace with the notion that consuming certain foods activates the body's natural slimming mechanisms. On top of that, this diet doesn't require giving up on chocolate and wine, which is one of its many perks.

What are the proven benefits of the Sirtfood diet? This diet has the potential to:

- **Stimulate your cells to repair and rejuvenate your body.** Consuming Sirtfoods, which will be explained in more detail later in the book, is linked with slowed aging, better metabolism, and improved circadian rhythm.
- **Regulate the metabolism of glucose and fat.** Sirtuins have been proven to regulate protein functioning by acting as a metabolic sensor. They were found to benefit overall health in both humans and animals. While there's still very little research to support the claim that sirtuins directly slow down aging, it's been confirmed that they contribute to longevity circumstantially by improving health and well-being in other ways.
- **Slow down aging.** Consumption of Sirtfoods create effects in your body that are similar to fasting and exercising. It can also help heal from the effects of eating junk food, as it includes foods rich in antioxidants that help detoxify your body. What's particularly appealing about this diet is that it includes dark

chocolate and red wine, making small dietary restrictions much easier to cope with.

- **Consuming Sirt foods will stimulate your sirtuin genes.** Sirtuin genes, which will be discussed in more detail throughout this book, boost your metabolism and help you burn fat. Due to their rejuvenating properties, sirtuins are often referred to as "longevity genes."
- **Sirt foods and the sirtuin proteins that they stimulate also affect your circadian rhythm.** The circadian rhythm is the cycle of physiological processes in all living beings that takes place for 24 hours. The circadian rhythm affects your health in numerous ways, mainly by regulating your sleep cycle, hormonal level, and most relevant for this topic—your appetite. However, this cycle can be disrupted by an unhealthy diet and lifestyle. Spending a lot of time in front of screens, eating unhealthy foods, and being sleep deprived can kick your hormones out of balance. This affects not only your appetite, but also your metabolism, mood, and overall mental state.

There is a reason why so many celebrities choose this diet. As it turns out, both Hollywood stars and regular folk have trouble introducing all the necessary changes that generate a fat loss simultaneously. Not only diet, but also the change in eating habits and regular exercise are difficult to apply to a busy lifestyle. Lack of time and money often gets in the way of doing your best, despite having the best of intentions.

While diet, exercise, and lifestyle changes all play a role in weight loss, the diet is the main factor. It gives you the strength and fuels your body with nutrients needed to work and exercise. Without the right diet, it's impossible to keep up with the rest of the changes needed for permanent weight loss.

The Sirtfood diet gives you all the convenience and satisfaction of a regular, healthy diet, but with a twist. It is tailored around a group of seven proteins called 'sirtuins' or SIRT proteins, that have been proven to extend lifespan, reduce inflammations, and boost metabolism. Eating Sirtfoods, however, won't feel very different compared to eating a regular, healthy diet. This is because the foods that increase your body's SIRT levels are quite plain and accessible to everyone. The natural compounds found in these foods help boost the sirtuin levels in your body, and the list includes the most mundane foods you can find in every grocery store, like kale, strawberries, parsley, onions, olive oil, walnuts, and others.

As you can see, there's nothing particularly special for you to do or eat to follow this diet. The diet includes two phases, the first being the most challenging, and second slightly easier. After completing the diet, you can choose between returning to your regular diet, or proceeding to eat Sirt Foods for as long as you want. There's no restriction for the amount of Sirt foods you can eat because all of them have healthy properties and are otherwise beneficial for your health. The creators of this diet ran a small pilot study, which showed that all of their participants lost over 7 lb while following the program (Goggins & Matten, 2017).

The study participants followed the Sirtfood diet program throughout 7 days. During this time, they lost an average of 3.2 kg without losing muscle mass. This is important because most fad diets cause initial weight loss, but not fat loss. This is because, when overly calorie deprived, our bodies first get rid of excess water, and then start burning muscle tissue to compensate for the lacking calorie supply. The information that study participants who followed the Sirtfood diet haven't lost any muscle mass is important because it indicates that the diet has, indeed, led to burning fat quite quickly.

However, it is also important to note that the recorded weight loss resulted from the diet's most challenging phases, which are phase one and two. Speedy weight loss can be explained with the fact that, when there's a lack of calories for your body to use, it uses its glycogen stores, as well as fat supplies. This way, during the first stage of the diet, your body will burn excess water, glycogen, and fat into the necessary energy to use. At this stage, a third of the weight lost will be from fat, while the remaining lost pounds will eventually come back after your body replenishes water and glycogen supplies.

While the first two stages of the diet serve to jump-start your metabolism, the third phase of the diet is the one to lead to actual permanent weight loss. As your metabolism is sparked due to the initial calorie restriction, you will now continue to supply your body with sirtuin boosting foods. Over time, the health benefits of the diet will build up, and you will experience a noticeable change in your health. The following section will further explain the recorded health benefits of the Sirtfood diet.

Well-Being Wonders

Now that you know what the Sirtfood diet is, it's time to learn a bit more about its health benefits. First things first, this diet doesn't require you to starve yourself or give up any food groups. Instead, this diet activates the production of sirtuin proteins with the use of carefully chosen foods to target fat loss while preserving your muscle mass.

The creators of the diet, Glen Matten and Aidan Goggins based their concept on the diets found in so-called Blue Zones, regions where people live exceptionally long. The Sirtfood diet creators concluded that one of the reasons for the longevity of the people inhabiting the Blue Zones lies in plant-rich diets that are particularly abundant in polyphenols (Goggins & Matten, 2017).

The diet typical for people living in Blue Zones is light, diverse, organic, and based on plants. This diet creates effects that are similar to fasting and thought to be behind the activations of sirtuin genes. In many ways, this diet is similar to the Mediterranean diet, which is confirmed to help prevent chronic illnesses. While this diet is fairly new, two key points are important to consider. First, the diet is shown to increase sirtuin levels. Second, sirtuin is found to help fat burning and improve sensitivity to insulin.

On the other hand, many of the recommended Sirt foods have been proven to yield important health benefits. Turmeric, green tea, and dark chocolate are certain to help reduce blood pressure and lower the risk of inflammations and heart disease. That is if you consume these foods in the recommended amounts and introduce all other recommended treatments and lifestyle changes. Studies also found that turmeric helps fight off chronic illnesses and inflammations if consumed consistently throughout a longer period.

The Sirtfood diet recommends the use of a few other 'superfoods.' These foods are found to have a powerful impact on human health and include green juice, buckwheat, lovage, and matcha green tea powder. During the first phase of the diet, when your calorie intake will be limited and you'll drink abundant doses of green juice, you will give your body a cleanse from toxins that have built up. Still, you will enjoy one delicious meal per day, which will consist mainly of Sirt foods.

One of the biggest benefits of this diet is that it helps you smoothly transition into a plant-based lifestyle. During the second phase of the diet, you'll increase your daily calorie intake and diversify the foods. This way, your diet remains versatile but clean and healthy. One of the major health benefits of this diet is that it helps you quit fats and sugars cold-turkey, and helps give them up completely by replacing them with flavorful meals and juices. This way, you gradually shift your eating habits and start eating clean. By phase three of the diet, which further increases your daily calorie intake and introduces even more Sirt foods, you will probably learn to satisfy your food cravings only using healthy plants.

Ultimately, you can continue reaping the health benefits of this diet long after its third week. While the first two phases serve you to lose weight, the third week of the diet teaches you how to permanently change your relationship with food. It incorporates all remaining Sirt foods into your regular diet, ensuring gradual but steady weight loss. You can start adding more Sirt foods into your usual recipes or replace some of the ingredients with the recommended Superfoods to increase the nutritional value and health benefits of your meals.

This way, the Sirtfood diet helps you gradually change your eating habits and overall relationship with food in a way that's simple and easy. This is particularly important because eating habits were found to be a significant factor behind all successful diets. While there are many diet plans, like the Keto diet, Intermittent fasting, and the balanced diet, that were found to result in long-term weight loss and health benefits, all of the researchers found that having a well-planned, steady eating schedule played a crucial role in maintaining progress. On the other hand, most of us find it difficult to give up old vices. The Sirtfood diet helps you do that with the use of strong-flavored foods that leave all of your senses satisfied.

On top of helping you change eating habits, this diet also helps jump-start your metabolism. As you start phase one and consume more healthy beverages like green tea that have been proven to reduce risks from heart disease and lower blood pressure, your body identifies that the sirtuin levels have increased, and starts to burn fat to compensate for the lacking calories. This way, you will lose fat directly, without diminishing your muscle mass. Some research indicates that sirtuins link with lower risk from Alzheimer's and heart disease. In animal studies, increased sirtuin levels are also linked with lower risks of developing tumors and cancer.

On top of this, the Sirtfood diet is one of the most accessible and easiest to follow diet programs out there that secure adequate nutrient balance. While there might be a lack of definite proof that sirtuin effects link to this particular diet, this plan certainly incorporates all elements necessary for permanent weight loss and long-term health and longevity. It acknowledges the necessity for adequate calorie intake (1,500 and higher during the third phase), flavor and abundance, and convenience of the diet to secure long-term effects. Aside from this, the diet secures adequate hydration with green juice and the elimination of sugary beverages. This way, you gradually train your body to stop craving sweets and instead get used to obtaining sugars from fruit and dietary fiber.

Now that you know about all the nutritional benefits of this diet, let's explain how it helps activate the so-called "skinny gene."

What Is the "Skinny Gene" and How to Activate It

The gene called SIRT 1 gene is linked with anti-aging effects, longevity, and disease prevention. Research discovered that the best way to activate this gene is through a healthy diet. Aside from activating your "Skinny gene," you also need to take good care of it to maintain its activity and experience the beneficial effects. Research showed that there are multiple strategies you can use to activate this gene. They all revolve around your diet, particularly around its timing and content (Kuningas et al., 2017).

SIRT 1 is a gene found both in humans and other mammalian animals. Its main role is to secure survival by providing cellular protection in conditions of food scarcity. Other animal species have similar genes as well, with a gene called SIR 2 being found in fruit flies, worms, and yeast. SIRT 1 acts protectively, and it prevents cells from dying by repairing damage caused by free radicals. It is also responsible for stimulating cellular mitochondria to produce more energy, helping extend lifespan and boost weight loss.

This gene also prevents fat in our bodies by being stored. It increases fat metabolism, resulting in storing smaller resources of fat in cells. This links to reduced risks from illnesses related to aging, cardiovascular diseases, osteoporosis, arthritis, and diabetes. All of these diseases are linked to excess fat stores inside one's body, and the reduction of these fat supplies also reduces the risks of diet-related diseases. This gene also links to slowed aging because of its anti-inflammatory and anti-oxidative properties. This means that SIRT 1 has the potential to reduce inflammations that lead to chronic illness, and it also prevents cellular oxidation that causes cells and tissues to age and die out prematurely.

But, all of these benefits only occur if you activate this gene using a couple of different strategies. Because SIRT 1 is protective, it will only activate if you reduce your calories and increase your activity levels. This way, you'll trigger protective mechanisms in your body that speed up metabolism to supply energy for your body and burn fat in the process. Aside from following the Sirtfood diet, there are also several other strategies that you can use to activate your skinny gene.

One of the strategies to activate your SIRT 1 gene is to eat less on certain days. Ideally, you'll eat your regular diet for five days of the week, and then reduce your intake of food for the remaining two days. This principle is similar to that present in the Paleolithic diet, which shares many staple foods with the Sirtfood diet. If you decide to reduce or limit calorie intake for two days of the week, you will still have to make sure to meet all of your nutritional needs and maintain the minimum calorie intake (1,000-1,500) for your body and mind to function properly. This principle was somewhat confirmed in some research studies that ran in the 1980s, which showed that animals who restricted their food intake occasionally but otherwise ate highly nutritious diets, lived longer and were healthier compared to those animals who ate constantly.

Exercise is another way to activate your skinny gene. Eating less while exercising more is a major lifestyle shift for someone who used to eat inconsistently and perhaps didn't work out at all. Here, you must balance your calorie intake to settle the minimum nutritional needs while exercising, but not more than the number of calories that you're consuming. Adding to that, finding a proper exercise routine that's suitable for your health, body type, and lifestyle is vital for optimum success. You should exercise a minimum of three times per week. Your workout routine should also be versatile to stimulate all muscle groups (Stefanick, 1993).

Eating foods rich in the substance called *resveratrol* will help sustain your energy levels as you eat less and exercise more (Lagouge et al., 2006).

Resveratrol is found in leafy greens, as well as citruses, mulberries, grapes, and high-quality wines. You can also consume this substance in the form of a supplement, in which case around 100 mg per day should be your target dose. Researchers from Harvard Medical School verified that there is indeed a connection between resveratrol and SIRT 1, confirming that the substance activated the skinny gene in their experimental yeast specimens. If taken in sufficient amounts, resveratrol will help you exercise more effectively while maintaining a lower calorie intake.

While eating the right foods can, indeed, potentially help activate the SIRT 1 gene, it's also important to keep in mind that the foods you eat need to be organic and come from quality produce. For example, red wine contains many substances said to activate SIRT 1, but this only applies to pure, organic red wine. Commercial wines can very well contain only a blend of artificial aromas and food colorings, which don't have any beneficial effects on your health, and they most certainly don't contribute to weight loss.

Summary

Great job! You've learned the basics of the Sirtfood diet and the science behind it. In this chapter, you found out that foods known to increase the levels of sirtuin protein link with:

- Improvements in overall health in longevity
- Regulation of blood glucose and blood pressure
- Long-term weight loss
- Lowering the risk and support in recovery from cardiovascular disease and metabolism-related diseases, like type 2 diabetes and insulin resistance.

You also found out that eating Sirtfoods indicates the activation of SIRT 1 genes that are linked with increased metabolism and longevity. You found out that a substance called *resveratrol*, found in the majority of foods recommended by the creators of the Sirtfood diet helps activate this gene, but it also helps one exercise more while eating fewer calories and preserving muscle mass in the process. This is particularly important because weight loss requires an initial investment of time and energy to restrict your calorie intake, but increase calorie expenditure and spark metabolic processes. Because this is quite hard and demanding for most people to do, diet is used as a way to supply substances that make it manageable and tolerable. Sirtfoods will aid the most demanding weight loss stage and keep you refreshed, energized, and feeling full, as you start to do the heavy work of creating daily calorie deficit. Now that you know the Basics of the Sirtfood diet, let's start learning how to apply it. The next chapter will provide tips for altering your diet and lifestyle to secure healthy weight loss.

Chapter 2:

Fighting Fat: How to Lose Fat in Best Possible Way With Sirtfood Diet

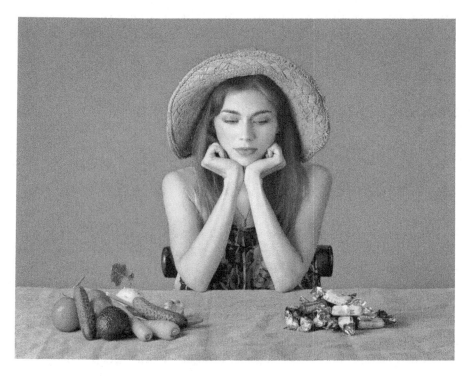

As you learned, the main challenge when going on any diet is to ensure a balanced nutrient intake, a steady daily calorie deficit, and an increase in daily calorie expenditure. Not easy for someone with an already strong appetite, right? Unless you design your diet well, you could easily end up with short-term muscle loss and nutrient deprivation. In this chapter, you'll learn about different aspects that play a role in permanent weight loss. You'll learn why fat loss is different from muscle loss, and how to use a Sirtfood diet to preserve muscles while burning fat. More importantly, you'll learn how the Sirtfood diet helps you change habits, and how unconscious and emotional eating relate with obesity and weight gain. With this knowledge, you'll be able to better monitor your habits, meals, and portion sizes.

In this chapter, you will also learn how to become an intuitive eater, and why this phrase isn't just a cliché from typical self-help books. You'll learn all about the organic, physiological background or eating intuition, how it may be affected by a poor diet, and more importantly, repaired with a healthy plant based diet. This will help you understand the urgency to quit junk food and start making sure that you've eaten as many Sirt Foods as possible in a single day.

Become a Master of Muscle

How Protein Helps Build Muscles

By now, you know that healthy weight loss means, among other things, eating sufficient protein to maintain or grow muscles while burning fat. For this, it is essential that you design a nutrient-rich, balanced diet that's abundant both in plants as well as meats and carbs. However, just increasing your protein intake doesn't guarantee muscle gain or maintenance. To spark the process of muscle growth, you need just the right amount of protein. Too much protein leads to dehydration, and too little won't prevent muscle loss while losing weight. If you're exercising, you will need 0.8 grams of protein per each kilogram of your weight daily.

As you already learned, one of the most important benefits of the Sirtfood diet is that it boosts fat burning while preserving or even growing muscle mass and reducing weight. In this section, we'll delve into this topic a bit deeper and explain how and why this happens, and what you can do to grow or maintain your muscle mass while losing weight. This information will not only help you design your diet but also understand which macronutrient ratio you want to maintain in your diet and what percentage of your meal will consist of Sirt foods for optimum muscle maintenance or growth.

The Sirtfood Diet for Those Who Work Out

Whether you're aiming mainly to reduce fat, or you're also trying to shape up and build your muscle mass, the knowledge of how much protein and fats you need is vital. It can make a difference between burning fat and noticing rock-solid abs showing on your belly, or seemingly losing weight on the scale without any visual progress in your physique and no health improvement. Sirtuin proteins can greatly assist in building muscle mass while burning fat. Recent research discovered a connection between muscle tissue regeneration and sirtuin protein levels. Essentially, higher sirtuin levels meant easier regeneration of the muscle tissue after it's been damaged during exercise.

What does this mean? As research findings indicate, sirtuin protein can potentially aid muscle tissue in its regeneration post-exercise and after injury. When you exercise, your muscles are put under strain, and tiny damages in their tissue form as a result. This is a reason why most of us suffer from muscle pain after exercise, particularly if we haven't been in good shape, to begin with. What you probably didn't know is that muscle mass is built when your body produces extra muscle cells and tissues to repair these tiny damages. Knowing that sirtuin proteins can help speed up or merely maintain this process is important to highlight the intake of Sirt foods if you're exercising.

Research also showed that sirtuin proteins may aid rejuvenation and recovery of heart muscle tissue as well, which is of particular significance for cardiovascular health. The more we age, the lesser the ability of our body to repair muscle damage. SIRT 1 has been shown to increase the speed and intensity of muscle function and repair in mice, increasing their muscle force significantly compared to the control group of test animals (the animals that didn't have increased SIRT 1 levels) (Chalkiadaki et al.,2014).

Another important fact to consider is that muscles don't only serve to help us move and generate strength. They also secrete cytokines and other biochemicals into our bloodstream, affecting other biological functions. In this sense, muscles play an important role in keeping the body well-balanced. When skeletal muscles function properly, they play a critical part in processing blood glucose. Sirtuins have been found to affect the regulation and metabolism of lipids and glucose. However, exercising causes metabolic stress to muscle cells in your body, leading to faster expending and consecutive production of sirtuin proteins. What does this mean?

While there are many ways to interpret research findings, it's safe to say that by consuming more sirtuin-boosting foods, you stimulate the production of the protein that enables healing and rejuvenation of your muscles. The more you exercise, the more you use up and further stimulate both your muscles and the sirtuin proteins, which is a chain reaction you can repeat over and over again to build your muscle mass. The more you exercise, the more sirtuin your body creates and uses to heal and regenerate muscles. As you learned in previous paragraphs, this means growing your muscle mass by creating microtears in their tissue and then harvesting the benefits of sirtuin to repair that tissue by growing more muscle cells.

Fat Loss VS Muscle Loss

Why is muscle maintenance important in weight loss? Unless your diet is designed to preserve your muscles, you can lose weight by 'burning' muscle tissue instead of fat. This way, you won't become healthier, mainly because your fat supplies will stay intact, or insufficiently reduced, affecting your health in the same negative way as if you hadn't lost weight at all. True, permanent weight loss means loss of fat. However, preserving muscle mass while losing weight is challenging for many reasons. First things first, muscles are built and preserved through lean protein intake. Although fats and carbohydrates have an important role in building muscle tissue and they shouldn't be eliminated from your diet; they should be significantly reduced to supply only the necessary energy without being stored in fat cells. Maintaining this ideal macronutrient ratio in meals isn't easy. It requires a lot of knowledge about portion sizes, composition (which proteins to eat and how much), and preparation (how to cook proteins to preserve them and how to use fats and oils in cooking while maintaining the right ratio).

Revamp Your Eating Habits

One of the things you learned so far is that the Sirtfood diet has one stand-out benefit, and that is helping you change your eating habits. As research shows, eating habits are vastly conditioned by the unconscious patterns we adopt through the influence of culture, our immediate surroundings, and the way we cope with feelings. Permanent weight loss, to a great extent, requires looking into these influences, identifying them, and deciding to change how we respond to them. The role of any diet plan, in this sense, is to provide a focus point for you to know your best dietary choices and to design meals to support health and weight loss while the more significant changes take place. This process is made a lot easier with the notion that there are 20 specific foods (which will be listed later on in this book) that you can turn to whenever you're hungry and need a snack. These foods are low in calories and rich in fiber and micronutrients (vitamins and minerals), and will be a great substitute for fast foods, starchy snacks, and sweets.

This is important because not only the exact foods you eat, but also the way in which you eat affects your health and chances of permanent weight loss. Significant weight loss and weight maintenance will require you to change your eating habits and adjust your environment to support healthy eating.

Your environment includes situations, settings, and people who affect the way you eat. Everything from your workspace to how you arrange your daily schedule, to how you set up your kitchen, pantry, and fridge can be used to support healthier eating. As you've probably noticed, the Sirtfood diet will require filling your fridge and pantry with abundant amounts of vegetables and organic spices, so that there's little to no space left for unhealthy foods. This way, when you get hungry, it will be easier to choose a serving of dates and strawberries instead of, let's say, Cheetos.

Changing your eating habits doesn't mean making huge changes in your lifestyle, but it does mean removing all the influences that contribute to irregular and unhealthy eating. The Sirtfood diet helps this process because it gives you an exact list of foods that support your health and weight loss that will be easy to implement in all of your meals. It will give you a simple, clean schedule for how you're supposed to eat.

Now let's discuss more how the composition of this diet helps you change your eating habits. The first phase of the diet will eliminate many fatty foods. As research shows, a healthy diet requires only small amounts of fat being eaten on a daily basis. The Sirtfood diet recommends eating abundant amounts of fruits and vegetables, which will keep you satisfied and full for the majority of the day.

Another way in which the search for the diet affects your eating habits is that it forces you to really be mindful about your meals, and portions. While it may look like eating in this way can be time consuming, it actually means that you are going to shift to focus on preparing foods in your home and in your kitchen. This eliminates the possibility, or reduces the temptations to order take out or eat out, where there are fewer healthy options to choose from. Aside from this, the Sirtfood diet also forces you to cook your meals, instead of eating premade meals or straight from the package. This helps control your portion size and meal composition. Last but not least, this diet helps you eat regularly and avoid skipping meals. Because Sirtfood meals are so easy to plan and prepare, you will be much less tempted to skip meals or eat larger meals at the end of the day. Here are a couple more common eating patterns that you'll overcome if you follow this diet:

How Sirt Foods Support Intuitive, Balanced Eating

To be an "intuitive eater" means to develop a strong connection with your body and look past all other influences (meal schedule, emotional eating, or cultural and societal expectations) and be aware of the foods your body truly needs for optimum nutrition and replenishment. This instinct gets skewed due to:

- The influences of sugar addiction that create strong and sudden cravings for unhealthy foods
- Eating to cope with overwhelming feelings
- Eating out of boredom, or
- Eating out of habit

During the first phase of the diet, you will experience a somewhat uncomfortable, but beneficial juice cleanse that will help you stop and shift the unconscious biological and mental processes that cause the previously mentioned behaviors. For a week, your diet will consist strictly of herbs, fruits, and vegetables, that will help balance your blood sugar and support the physiological processes that affect appetite to balance out.

How Sirt Foods Help Eliminate Bad Eating Habits

Introducing Sirt Foods into your diet will contribute to correcting some of the following unconscious behaviors that contribute to weight gain:

- **Habitual Eating**

Habitual eating is a behavioral pattern of having your meals because it's the appropriate time of the day, even if you're not hungry, or having certain (usually too large) amounts of food because you think that's how your meal should look. Overall, habitual eating contributes to eating too much and too frequently because you believe that's how you're supposed to eat, completely disregarding your actual appetite and the nutritional needs of your body. Correcting habitual eating is commonly done by paying more attention to whether or not you're truly hungry and becoming more aware of where your cravings and food choices come from. Essentially, correcting habitual eating means becoming more aware of the genuine, physiological appetite that arises when your body becomes depleted of energy.

The Sirtfood diet helps you do this with the introduction of fiber and vitamin-dense foods that replenish your intestinal flora. As research shows (Niccolai et al., 2019), health and biodiversity of your microbiome greatly affects your appetite and cravings through the connection known as the gut-brain axis. This neurological connection affects when you'll feel hungry and what you'll crave.

When your microbiome is healthy, the gut-brain axis 'communicates' your nutritional needs more efficiently. It enables your digestive system to signal when you need protein (meats), fat, or vegetables to supply a certain type of fuel to your body. But, when your microbiome is damaged, which happens when you eat too much unhealthy foods, this connection becomes disrupted, and you're no longer aware of true nutritional needs. Instead, when you spend your caloric reserves during the day, sugar addiction prevails, and you crave fried foods and sweets instead of lean meats and vegetables.

The best, and some would say, only way to recover from this digestive damage, is to go on a plant-based diet that will help grow the healthy bacteria inside your gut. If you look into the list of recommended foods to replenish your gut microbiome, you will notice that this list mostly consists of foods recommended in this book, with an addition of probiotics and prebiotics you get when you eat fermented foods.

The more you eat a plant-based diet, the more you're aware of how much meat, veggies, and sugar from organic fruits your body needs. This way, you eat in a way that supports the replenishment of your body and burning those stubborn fatty supplies from problematic areas.

- **Speed-Eating**

Speed-eating is a habit of eating on-the-go or by your kitchen counter as you rush to get through the day. It is harmful because it causes you to eat hundreds of calories more during the day than you actually need. As research shows, you only need around 100 extra calories during a day, which equals one small snack, to consistently gain weight. This is because these calories won't be spent during your daily activities, and will eventually be stored in fat cells.

Research also shows (Horwath et al., 2019) that you need to eat a meal for at least 20-30 minutes for your body to detect that you've eaten and start to send satiety signals. This is important because speed eating means eating your entire meal in ten minutes or less, making it more difficult for your body to detect when you've had enough food. This causes overeating, as you're able to eat more calories than you need without feeling full. How does the Sirtfood diet help correct this? The answer is simple.

Following the principles of this diet requires you to take the time and think through your meals in advance and invest time in cooking. It eliminates the rush out of the process and actually makes you set aside between 30 minutes and an hour to make and eat your meals. Aside from this, Sirtfoods are strong in flavor and more satiating than many of their alternatives. Strong flavors (Maier et al., 2017) are found to induce a sensation of satiety more quickly and intensely than less flavorsome foods, like deep-fried meat, for example.

To sum up, eating Sirt Foods helps you eat slower, more thoughtfully, and feel full with having eaten smaller quantities of food.

• Emotional and Cultural Eating

Cultural influences affect your choice of dishes and the manner of cooking, while feelings you associate with eating affect how much and how frequently you'll eat. These two types of influences intertwine (Waller & Matoba, 1999) and can completely alter one's diet to stem away from healthy eating and individual needs. Culturally speaking, most people learn to prepare foods in certain ways, oftentimes with more fat and oil being used than needed, and more dishes prepared for the sake of nurturing a warm, welcoming home environment. For many individuals and families, this means cooking in advance and more than you need so that you can have a fully set table at dinner time, often featuring dishes that are carb and fat-saturated. Most of us never question these cultural influences, but instead feel compelled to maintain this warm and welcoming vibe. While this doesn't apply to most people, for some, it can just mean too much available food to eat when you don't really need to eat, further contributing to weight issues.

Emotional eating, on the other hand, means eating under the influence of guilt and shame associated with refusing a meal, or to calm down and feel more emotionally satisfied in the absence of other, healthy, coping mechanisms. Emotional eating originates in childhood, when food is used abundantly to ensure that the child is well-fed, with emotional conditioning, like using guilt or fear, is used in situations when a child refuses to eat. Essentially, this means that, when you were a child, your caregivers were greatly concerned over whether you're eating enough. If you refuse to eat, they are afraid that you won't develop health or that you'll get sick, so they tell you things like "You have to eat to be healthy," or they make you feel guilty for refusing food when there's so much hunger in the world.

Adding to that, food is often used in childhood to help upset children calm down. Even worse, the foods that parents and caregivers most often use to soothe upset children include snacks and sweets. This is the main reason why so many people resort to candy and ice cream when they feel sad or bored. If you think about it, one of the easiest ways to distract a child who is crying or being overly active is to give them their favorite candy. Indeed, parents can get excruciatingly tired, but by doing this, they prevent their child (possibly you) from learning how to process stress and calm down on their own.

Considering the obesity rates worldwide, it's safe to say that most people find it difficult to abandon these childlike habits, even when they affect their health. Luckily, just by becoming aware of this, you can start looking for healthier ways to process difficult feelings. The Sirtfood diet, on the other hand, helps support this change by introducing tasty, satisfying foods you can turn without jeopardizing your health. The first week of the diet gives you a simple schedule to follow, and the recommended foods are designed to boost your energy and mood so that you don't crave sweets even if your day doesn't go well, and you feel down.

- **Binge-Eating**

Binge-eating can be both an occasional habit, or a full-blown eating disorder, depending on its frequency and impact on your health. Binge-eating is a behavior, or a behavioral pattern, of eating large portions of food at once for psychological reasons. For some people, it is a habit they can shake off with some awareness and training, while for others, it can become an eating disorder that requires months of therapy to recover from. Binge-eating is harmful because it not only contributes to obesity (studies show that two-thirds of obese people have this disorder), but also because it worsens anxiety and prevents people from coping with stress, fear, and sadness in healthy ways. How does the Sirtfood diet help prevent and support recovery from binge eating?

The answer is simple. The foods that boost your sirtuin levels are also proven to stabilize mood (McClung, 2013) because they contain healthy fiber and vitamins that have shown to lower stress hormones and boost the serotonin levels. You probably know that serotonin is also called "happiness hormone," and that it helps you feel calmer, happier, and overall more emotionally balanced. The more you include Sirt foods into your diet, the better and more emotionally stable you'll feel over time.

- **Crash Dieting**

Crash-dieting is a habit of going on short-term, highly restrictive diets to lose weight quickly, and then re-gaining the weight as soon as you stop following the restrictive diet. Crash-dieting usually consists of minimizing your daily calorie intake to less than 1,000 calories per day, which is below what's needed for your body to function properly. Doing this over a short amount of time causes your body to use its water reserves for basic functioning, and can result in losing 5-10 lb over only a couple of days. While this result may lead you to think that you've lost weight, and that weight loss will persist in weeks to come, the weight usually bounces back the moment you stop restricting calories and replenish the water reserves in your body.

While the Sirtfood diet does begin with a week-long juice cleanse, and it does restrict your calorie intake to 1,000 calories during the first, and 1,500 calories during the second week, it consists of foods that supply your body with hydration and proteins. This was proven in the study done by the diet creators (Goggins & Matten, 2017), that showed that those who followed the program, and even exercised intensely during the most restrictive period of the diet, have, in fact, lost fat instead of water weight. On top of that, they maintained their muscle mass, which isn't typical for those who crash-diet.

The second reason why weight loss with the Sirtfood diet is consistent is that the first phase of the diet is followed by a gradual, systematic, and healthy calorie increase during the second phase. During the second week of the diet, you will increase your calorie intake to 1,500, but you will do so in a lean, nutrient-dense way. Your meals will consist mainly of nutrient-packed vegetables, lean meats, and healthy, organic carbs, that will all instantly supply your body with nutrients needed for you to be in a good mood, energized, and sharp-minded. While the diet you follow gives you instant fuel to function properly, your body will then spend another seven days shifting from burning blood glucose to burning fat. This shift is crucial for jump-starting metabolism.

One of the reasons why stubborn fat supplies are so hard to get rid of is that you haven't yet trained your body to use these supplies. With the increase of sirtuin protein levels, you'll be able to exercise more while eating less, leaving your body with no other option than to burn fat. I'll argue many times throughout this book that one of the biggest benefits of this diet is that it supports your body in switching from using blood glucose as an immediate fuel to burning fat. This was also confirmed by many research studies that showed that a plant based diet, in addition to exercise, hydration, and quality sleep, helps trigger constant and even fat burning.

Last, but not least, the Sirtfood diet is highly sustainable. The plan is easy to follow, and you don't have to calorie-restrict past the second week of the diet. How will this support your weight loss? The answers are simple here as well. During the first weeks of the diet, you will learn to eat in a way that's centered around your body and health, and not habits, culture, feelings, and mood. You will become aware of how this manner of eating compares to your previous eating patterns and be better able to control what and how much you eat. The healthy foods you'll eat during this time will supply your body with vitamins and minerals, and your metabolism will shift to burning fat. Once you no longer have to restrict your calories, you'll know how to measure your portions to avoid overeating, and the constant intake of sirtuin-boosting foods will further support fat burning and muscle growth.

In this chapter, you learned about all the proven benefits of the Sirtfood diet. You learned how this diet will affect your body on the inside, by triggering your metabolism, and on the outside, by helping you develop awareness for healthy eating. In the next chapter, you'll learn about the exact steps needed to follow this diet and the foods needed throughout the process.

Chapter 3:

The Sirtfood Diet: The Best 20

Sirtfoods

Now that you know the basic postulates and the scientific explanations behind the Sirtfood diet, it's time to learn how to apply the concept so that you too can lose weight permanently. First things first, your diet will consist of the so-called "Sirt foods" that activate and boost the levels of sirtuin in your body. If you shape your diet around the top Sirt foods mentioned below, you will quickly and easily boost your health and metabolism and reduce inflammation. The foods that will be included in your daily meals are the following:

- **Bird's-eye chili peppers** are known for their weight-loss-friendly properties. They can increase your metabolism and body temperature, hence boosting your metabolism rates. They are also helpful to improve your digestion and prevent fat from accumulating in your body.
- **Buckwheat** is another superfood used in the Sirtfood diet. Its health benefits are numerous, as it has proven antioxidant and high mineral content that helps control blood sugar. Aside from being nutrient-dense, buckwheat also contains plenty of protein. However, keep in mind that it's mainly made of carbohydrates when planning your meals. It is rich in manganese, copper, magnesium, iron, and phosphorus, which are all nutrients you can easily become deprived of when you follow calorie-restricted diet plans.

- **Capers** have amazing benefits for your overall health, but particularly for your skin and hair. If you follow recipes given in this book, you'll mainly use them to garnish and season your meals. Rutin, a compound found in capers, is a powerful antioxidant that helps improve blood circulation and the health of your blood vessels. Quercetin, another potent antioxidant found in this plant, has anti-carcinogenic, antibacterial, anti-inflammatory, and analgesic properties.

- **Celery** is abundant in potent antioxidants that protect your cells and blood vessels. It contains flavonoids, beta carotene, vitamin C, and 12 more antioxidants that protect against inflammations. Aside from this, celery supports the health of your digestive tract as it helps prevent harmful bacteria from overpopulating.

- **Cocoa**, one of the staple foods in this dietary concept, is proven to contain antioxidants like polyphenols, that help fight off infections and inflammations, improve blood circulation, lower blood cholesterol, and control blood sugar.

- Despite being commonly banished from the majority of popular diet plans, **coffee** helps lower blood sugar and is said to help prevent illnesses like diabetes, Parkinson's, Alzheimer's, and cancer. However, too much coffee can cause anxiety, and even lead to panic attacks. While you can have coffee on the Sirtfood diet, make sure to have it earlier in the day and only in amounts that don't affect your mood negatively.

- **Extra virgin olive oil** is abundant in antioxidants and healthy fats. Research showed that consuming small amounts of extra virgin olive oil each day helps prevent heart disease. Ideally, you'll have around 1.5 tbsp of this oil daily. However, make sure to purchase top quality oil because regular olive oil doesn't contain any of the aforementioned healthy fats, and is proven to clog arteries.

- **Matcha green tea** links to many health benefits, including stimulation of weight loss, cancer prevention, prevention of type 2 diabetes, and heart diseases. These properties are attributed to the epigallocatechin gallate (EGCG). The optimum dose of this tea is up to two servings per day, which can be translated into 10 to 20 cups of regular green tea. Since there's a maximum recommended daily amount, you should pay attention not to exceed this dose when making your daily green juice and using matcha green tea in your meals.
- **Lovage** is best known for its digestive properties. It's confirmed to help relieve stomach discomfort and gas, but it also helps cardiovascular health. Because it acts as a diuretic, it's considered to have a purifying effect on the blood and helpful in treating kidney stones. Because of its intense flavor, it's often used in small amounts to season soups, meats, and vegetables.
- **Kale** is considered a superfood because a single cup of this chopped vegetable contains over 100% of recommended daily intake of vitamins A, C, and K. It is also abundant in copper, potassium, and manganese, which are all vital for the maintenance and optimum functioning of your immune system. Kale is confirmed to be helpful in fighting off cancer in raw and cholesterol in steamed form, which indicates that you should aim to cook it on the lowest possible temperatures and as briefly as possible to reap the most benefits.
- **Parsley** is rich in antioxidants and proven to support bone health, contains substances that help maintain your eye health and prevent cancer, supports and improves cardiovascular health, fights off bacterial infections, and helps weight loss. One of the greatest advantages of parsley is that it's easy to include in almost all cooked meals. It will taste great in soups, salads, and meats and other vegetables. However, eating too much parsley may cause allergic reactions. For this reason, aim

to stick to the highest recommended daily dose of a maximum of ten springs.

- **Medjool dates,** while known as quite a sweet fruit, are actually low in sugar but abundant in fiber. Due to their composition, they will keep you energized for a long time without increasing your blood sugar. They are a useful snack while dieting because they're sweet, tasty, and satiating, but don't cause blood glucose to spike as other sugar-dense foods do.

- **Red chicory** is another fiber-dense food that is useful to support digestion. Because it is prebiotic, it will support the health of your gut bacteria. Gut bacteria directly correlate to metabolic and immune system functioning. Using it regularly will help gently suppress appetite and control cravings. It will help prevent constipation and relieve gas. Aside from this, chicory is also known to be a powerful oxidant and possess anti-inflammatory properties. If you take it regularly, it will also help regulate your heart rate, prevent cancer, and support the health of your liver and gallbladder.

- **Red wine,** organic and high quality varieties, contain antioxidants that promote longevity and boost your immune system. Pinot Noir is considered to have the highest concentration of beneficial compounds. However, make sure to limit your daily intake to one glass. Drinking too much wine can be possibly unsafe and cause mood swings. While an average dose of one glass of red wine per day supports weight loss, excess amounts will actually cause weight gain. While on the Sirtfood diet, and particularly if you're on a busy schedule that dictates being active and focused for a significant portion of the day, it might be best to drink wine in the evening or before going to bed.

- **Red onion** is shown to support heart health as it contains potent antioxidants. If you eat regular doses of red onions, you'll reduce cholesterol and decrease triglycerides and inflammations. The anti-inflammatory properties in this vegetable are linked with decreased risks from many chronic illnesses, and particularly from heart disease. Too much onion can cause nausea and bloat, so make sure to keep your daily intake at recommended daily dosage. While this vegetable is the healthiest raw, most people find its taste too overwhelming. When cooking onions, avoid exposing them to high temperatures for longer than three minutes, as this might kill off the majority of their healthy nutrients.

- **Strawberries** are packed with antioxidants, fiber, vitamin C, and other nutrients. They are proven to support cardiovascular health, improve good (HDL) cholesterol, prevent cancer, and regulate blood pressure. However, you should aim to have a maximum of eight strawberries per day. Too many, and you might have an allergic reaction. Also, like all other fruits, strawberries are sugar-dense and might spike your blood glucose levels if eaten in high amounts. When cooking according to your Sirtfood diet plan, aim to add a couple of fresh strawberries to your desserts and breakfast smoothies and porridges. Avoid cooking because high temperatures will kill off the majority of their beneficial nutrients.

- **Rocket**, or arugula, is another commonly known superfood. You can add It to green juices, salads, and smoothies to boost their nutritional value. Arugula is rich in vitamins E, C, K, and B and abundant in beta carotenes, chlorophyll, and amino acids. On top of that, it is also rich in glucosinolates, which are known to protect cancer.

- **Soy** is a satiating food that contains numerous vitamins and minerals. However, it has earned a negative reputation due to industrial cultivation and the use of pesticides. If you purchase only clean, organic soy, you will boost your plant protein intake. This will help regulate blood pressure and keep your cholesterol in check.

As you can see, there will be plenty of treats for you to enjoy on this diet! Unlike most diets that discourage consumption of coffee and alcohol, this one will allow you plenty of flexibility when participating in social events. You won't be the only person not to drink anything or have a tasty snack, and you'll also have plenty of options to unwind with at the end of a hard day.

During the first week of the diet, you will limit your calories to only 1,000 per day. This might be difficult, but noticing that 7 lb initial weight loss will surely help maintain your drive. On the plus side, you will be eating delicious meals and drinking plenty of satiating juices, which will make things easier. Aside from limiting your calorie intake, you will prepare three green juice mixes each day. The third rule is to also have one meal each day that's rich in Sirt foods.

Main phase: 7 lb in Seven Days: Is It Possible?

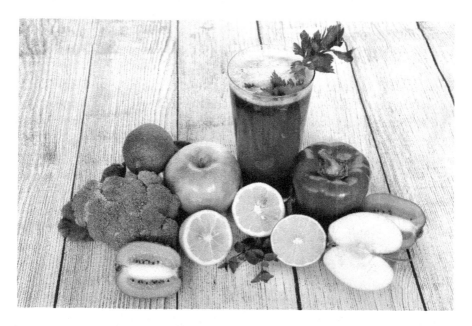

As you know by now, Sirtfood Green Juice is a staple meal of this diet concept. Juicing is a popular method used to spark calorie burning, but choosing the right greens for the juice can make a difference between kick-starting fat loss and dehydration and slowing down metabolism. If you wondered why it's important to determine, take a look at these two currently proven facts:

- Dieting with the use of Green juice ensured fat loss and muscle preservation with the use of Sirtfoods.
- Excessive juicing is proven to lead to muscle loss and yo-yoing.

But, how are both of these conflicting facts possible?

To answer that, let's address the main issue with juice dieting. Calorie deprivation that happens once all fiber is removed from the juice, doesn't provide sufficient nutrition for your body (this is why phase 1 includes one Sirtfood meal). To make the matters worse, those practicing juicing often go on days-long juice cleanses that last anywhere from three to 14 days. This is an excessively long time for your body to spend with no macronutrient intake. Remember, despite our not liking the fact that they feed fat cells, macronutrients are vital for the functioning of internal organs, including heart, liver, and kidney. How we use them is another story though.

When you go on a complete juice diet, you are sabotaging weight loss. It severely depletes you of calories, which will cause your metabolism to slow down, as it detects that your body is starving. When little to no calories are consumed, the human body triggers the same physiological mechanisms that take place if we get lost in the woods, or we don't have any available food. Calorie depletion is a red flag to your body that you're at risk of dying. In this situation, you may burn through glycogen supplies that often carry water, and quickly lose a couple of pounds as a result. This might boost your confidence temporarily, but the weight will come back as soon as you start eating regular foods again.

Unless done right, juicing can cause nutrient deprivation. You may not think this is possible since you're consuming large amounts of squeezed fruits and vegetables. But, remember, you're not eating any proteins, fats, and carbohydrates. On top of that, vitamin B12 deficiency is also present in those who juice for an extended period.

But, what if juicing could be used to spark metabolism? As you remember, the participants in the Sirtfood diet's creators didn't dehydrate, lose muscle mass, or become nutrient deficient. How did that happen? The answer lies in two important elements:

- The composition of the Sirtfood Green Juice
- The fact that you will eat one solid meal each day

With your daily meal, if well-balanced, you will consume enough macronutrients to keep your metabolism running. The potent mix that goes into the Sirt Juice will increase sirtuin levels, which will give your metabolism a boost, and temporarily restricted calories will create a daily calorie deficit, causing more calories to be burned. All of these influences, when combined, create ideal conditions for fat burning.

If you're afraid that phase 1 will slow down your metabolism or cause nutrient deprivation, don't worry. This won't happen because the solid foods you'll eat will supply enough fat, protein, and carbs for your metabolism to work, and the juice will influence it to work faster.

For this process to work, you should also base your solid meals on Sirtfoods, and make sure to have minimum recommended amounts of daily protein, carbs, and fat.

During the first week of the diet, you should drink three doses of Green Juice per day. During the first three days, you will have only one Sirtfood meal. After that, you will have two juices and two meals during the next four days. Here's how to make a serving of the Sirtfood Diet Green Juice:

You will need:

- 75 g or two handfuls of Kale
- 30 g of rocket
- 5 g of parsley, flat-leaf
- 5 g of lovage leaves
- 150 g of green celery with leaves
- One half of an apple
- Juice squeezed from one half of a lemon
- ½ tsp of matcha green tea

Steps:

- Juice mixed lovage, parsley, rocket, and kale. If necessary, re-juice to extract the maximum out of leafy greens because some juicers tend to have trouble with these plants. You should have around 50 ml after juicing. Optionally, if your juicer can't produce this amount, increase the dosage of the ingredients proportionally to achieve extra amounts.

- After that, juice your celery and apple half. Peel the lemon and run it through the juicer if you wish, but it might be easier to squeeze it beforehand and add it to the mix. This will increase the juice volume to 250 ml or even more. After this, add your matcha green tea.
- To mix in the matcha green tea, add it to the glass and stir until it's fully integrated into the juice. Use this ingredient for only two juices per day. Add the rest of the juice once the tea powder has dissolved.

Second Phase: The Secret to Maintenance Effects

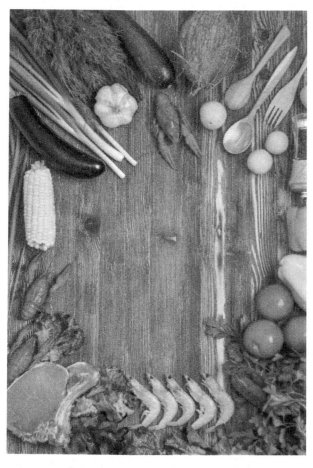

During the second phase of the diet, you will increase your calorie intake to 1,500. You will have two Sirtfood Green Juices each day and two meals rich in Sirt foods. During this phase, the biggest challenge will be to measure and design your meals to conform with the calorie limit, but still have a balanced macronutrient intake. On the plus side, the phase 2 of the Sirtfood diet doesn't require excluding fats, meats, and carbs. You will have all the freedom to eat any foods you want as long as you have enough SirtFoods incorporated in the menu. In this book, you'll find a large number of recipes for different diets, from carnivore to vegan, that you can use as your guide.

Eating a 1,500-calorie diet will create a significant daily calorie deficit. The amount of calories you otherwise spend daily depends on your lifestyle, activity levels, age, and gender. Accordingly, the amount of weight loss you can expect on a 1,500-calorie diet depends on how much calorie deficit will be created throughout phase 2. Keep in mind that, depending on your average daily calorie needs, this restriction may be more or less difficult. If your daily expenditure is somewhere around 1800 calories, you may not feel that substantial of a difference. But, if you burn more than 2000 calories daily, you can start to feel not only hungry but also dizzy or fatigued. While 1,500 per day won't harm your health short-term, there's a possibility of being energy-depleted unless you balance your meals well.

Your daily calorie expenditure can be accurately measured using the Mifflin-St Jeor equation, which accounts for weight, height, and age. The aforementioned equation is done by multiplying your weight ten times, adding your height multiplied by 6.25, and deducting five times your age number. Men will then add five to the result, and women will deduct 161. The resulting number states how many calories on average you burn daily.

However, this equation doesn't account for daily activity fluctuations. You will burn more calories on the days when you're more active, and less when you're resting, working in the office, and not working out. This is important to consider both during phase 2 and the maintenance. In this phase of the diet, more activity will create a larger calorie deficit, which may or may not yield greater weight loss. For this reason, the equation accounts for five different types of lifestyle by activity levels. If you lead a sedentary lifestyle, you'll multiply your score by 1.2, and 1.375 if you're lightly active. Moderately active individuals should multiply their score by 1.55, very active by 1.725, and extra active people, or those who exercise intensively twice or more per day, will multiply their score by 1.9.

You will have to keep this in mind when measuring your meal portions during the maintenance phase. Usually, more active days require a boost of protein and carbs, while being less active requires a greater ratio of vegetables and fruits compared to meat and carbs.

Regardless of individual differences in daily calorie expenditure, a daily deficit of 500 calories is thought to be safe and help you lose at least 1 pound per week. If this weight loss grade was accurate, most people would lose up to 55 lb yearly. But, many other psychological, health, and lifestyle factors affect one's ability to lose weight consistently. Stress, lack of knowledge, and the ability to balance macronutrients in your meal, lack of resources to purchase quality foods, and others, are recognized as being a cause for significantly reducing weight loss rates.

In these circumstances, Sirtfoods play an important role. They help you maintain this desired calorie deficit because they're affordable and more available compared to other foods used in weight loss studies. To boost your chances of permanent weight loss, the first, and most important task, is to design your diet so that you eat mainly whole foods, and organic and lean fats and protein.

Now, onto the big questions: How and what should you actually eat during the second phase to be well-nourished and to feel good? If we know that carb (+ fiber-rich veggies): protein: fat should be 50%: 25%: 25%, that means that you should design your meals to include:

- Carbohydrate, 750 calories
- Protein, 350 calories and
- Fats, 350 calories

Sounds easy, does it? But, when you're supposed to figure out how to make your breakfast, lunch, and dinner to conform within these limits, and account for the small amount of calories gained from Sirt Green Juice, things may start to get confusing. Let's break down how your daily meal plan should look during phase 2:

- Sirtfood Green Juice, 2 servings 180 calories (90 calories each)

- Breakfast, lunch, and dinner, approx. 440 calories for each meal. This will then mean 200 calories worth of carbs, 120 calories worth of protein, and 12o calories in fat per each meal.

While being on a 1,500 calorie diet is said to be overly restrictive, it doesn't have to be that way if you pay attention to what you're eating. Compared to an average, unmonitored diet, you could easily end up eating more nutritious foods than if you ate 2,000 calories of saturated fats and unhealthy carbs, with little to no fruits and vegetables. On the other side of the spectrum is the fact that you can be both obese and nutrient-deprived at the same time, much like how you can be skinny but still have too much fatty tissue.

Now that you know what calorie distribution on the Sirtfood diet should look like, let's talk more about what you can do to boost your sirtuins permanently, once you're done with the diet program.

Phase Three: Sirtfood for Life

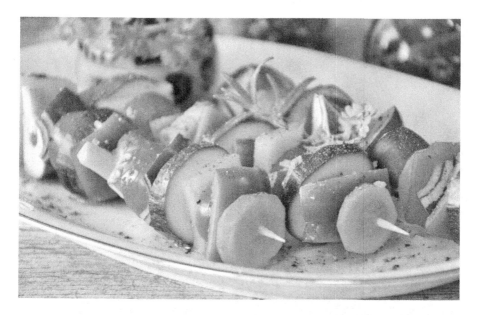

After you've completed the second phase of the diet, you will work to adjust your meals and lifestyle to eat as many Sirt foods as you can daily. This diet has helped many celebrities, including Sir Ben Ainslie, Lorraine Pascale, and Jodie Kidd to lose weight. One of the biggest benefits of this diet is that your nutrient intake will be extremely high. All the foods included in the diet plan are rich in fiber, minerals, and vitamins that will undoubtedly replenish your body and boost your immune system. However, you should keep in mind that the first week of the diet will eliminate many food groups, which might affect your energy levels and ability to focus. With that in mind, schedule the beginning of your diet so that the first days don't fall on those days of the week when you expect to be active the most. You should also avoid going on this diet if you have diabetes or if your lifestyle is active and intense. The first week of the diet might bring some headaches or a light-headed feeling before your body gets used to lower calorie intake.

Secrets Tips to Sirtfood Cooking and Long-Term Weight Maintenance

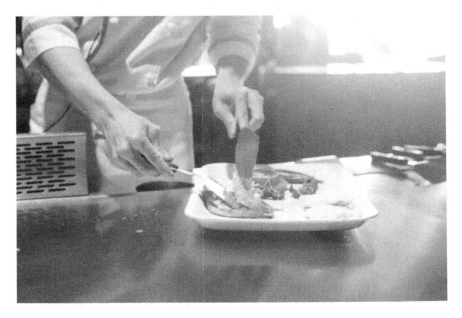

After you've lost initial weight and set the grounds for building healthy eating habits, the final stage on your weight loss journey will require you to learn how to maintain your weight loss and cook your Sirt Foods properly.

First things first, long-term weight loss maintenance will require doing everything you can to prevent the weight from coming back. This poses a challenge for nearly 85% of those who lose weight. The reasons for this is that decreasing the calorie intake in order to lose weight may lead to reducing metabolic rates in the months to come. Returning to a 'normal' diet increases your average calorie intake, increasing the chances of gaining the weight back. This is the main reason why long-term calorie restriction isn't recommended and why you need to focus on losing weight slowly and consistently. As such, focusing on a long-term healthy eating regimen, aside from eating as many Sirt Foods as possible, ensures that you won't return to harmful habits of habitual, speed, and emotional eating. After you've completed the first two weeks of the Sirtfood diet, you should focus on the following strategies to keep the weight off:

Diet and exercise planning. Studies show that those who manage to maintain an average of 1,500-2,000 calories per day and exercise daily, but not too intensely, achieve best results with long-term weight maintenance. This will require creating a loose and flexible diet plan, in which you'll calculate the desired daily calorie intake and list the foods you want to eat daily and weekly.

While you'll find more information on portion sizing and portion control in following sections, the first step to maintain your weight will be to gradually add no more than 200 calories of Sirtfoods to your daily menu. This means that you should increase your daily calorie intake to 1,700 calories in the first week, 1,900 calories during the second, and ultimately to 2,000-2,100 calories in the third week after completing the first two stages of the diet.

Mindfulness and awareness. Knowing how much unconscious factors, influences, and behaviors contribute to weight gain, you should keep track of your progress and eating patterns to see if environmental and emotional influences are again starting to affect your eating. Doing so will help you to be more aware of how you respond to stress and process daily struggles to avoid stress-eating. Doing everything you can to stay emotionally balanced, by practicing mindfulness techniques like journaling, meditation, and art, will help process daily difficulties in a healthier way, and more importantly, without eating.

Healthy lifestyle. As you already know, your weight isn't only conditioned by your diet. Stress affects your digestive health, as well as contributes to sleep deprivation. Paying attention to eating healthy, measured, and timely meals, will contribute to not only physical, but also psychological health and balance. Aside from supporting a healthy mind using Sirtfoods, you should also pay attention to shelter yourself from stress and becoming too overwhelmed. A mindful work schedule, careful time management, and enough time for healthy, relaxing physical activity, will help develop mental resilience to stress. The more balanced you are, the better you'll protect your digestive health. Remember, stress harms your hormonal balance and gut flora, which, in return, depletes your immune system, increases blood cholesterol and spikes your blood glucose. Consequently, you could start gaining weight back every time you become overwhelmed by stress.

Control your portion size. As you've noticed, chances of permanent weight loss increase with your ability to accurately measure your meals. Only a couple of extra spoonfuls a day can create a caloric surplus, and contribute to weight gain over time. For this reason, you should use the following strategies to better control your portion sizes:

Use the right-size plates and bowls. Measuring the exact amounts of meats, vegetables, and carbs to eat in a single meal guarantees a balanced diet. However, doing this with every meal isn't easy. Finding plates and bowls that match your recommended food quantities will help measure your portions. Studies showed that those who ate from large plates ate between 14% and 77% more food than those who ate from smaller plates, so keep that in mind when choosing your dinnerware.

Divide your plate to distribute foods. If you've chosen a right-sized plate that tightly fits your desired calorie intake, you can create a visual or a mental map of how to divide its surface to place different foods. For example, a rough guide on macronutrient ratios recommends to fill half of your plate with a salad or veggies (ideally Sirtfoods), one-fourth of your plate with protein, including meat, fish, poultry, eggs, dairy, pulses, and/or beans, one-fourth of complex carbs (pasta, potatoes, whole grains, etc.,) and a half of a tablespoon (up to seven grams) of high fat, like butter, cheese, and oils. Looking into this guide, spontaneous weight gain despite best efforts may start to make sense. Most of us, habitually, fill our plates with at least half carbs, not to mention the generous cheese portions most of us enjoy. As you can see, paying attention to how much of each food group you eat can make a substantial difference in carb and fat intake, and significantly affect weight maintenance.

Start small and build up. Whenever you're unsure of how much food to put on your plate, start with half. A half of a portion, when eaten slowly and over the course of at least 15 minutes, will be a good guide for how much more you want (or don't want) to eat. Furthermore, a smaller portion will prevent overeating as you won't feel compelled to finish the entire plate. This is particularly important when you're eating out, because restaurant serving sizes can be as twice as large compared to recommended serving sizes!

Preserve nutrients when cooking. Sirtfoods are all plants and vegetables, and you won't increase your sirtuin levels unless you cook these foods in a way that preserves their nutrients. This is particularly difficult because fibers, vitamins, and minerals found in vegetables dissolve in water and under the influence of heat. Ideally, eat as much raw vegetables as possible. When cooking, pay attention not to use too much water. Water will drain the vitamins from your Sirt veggies, particularly vitamins C and B. To retain maximum vitamins, steam and microwave vegetables instead of boiling. Particularly, avoid blanching leafy greens, beans, kale, and other vegetables, because this will destroy almost all of their nutrients. After you've cooked your vegetables, don't rush to cool them. Sudden temperature changes also affect nutrients. Set your dish aside instead of cooling with ice or putting it in the fridge, and eat it once it's cooled down at room temperature. Using fats thoughtfully, ideally in the form of extra virgin olive oil, will help the absorption of vitamin K, beta carotene, and vitamin D from your Sirt veggies. Topping your vegetables with citrus fruit juice, up to a spoonful, will add the vitamin C, which helps absorb iron found in leafy greens and almost all Sirt foods.

The following chapters (4-7) will give you recipes based on the original *"The SirtFood Diet"* recipes (Goggins & Matten, 2017), but altered and designed to be more versatile, simpler, and easier to make.

Chapter 4:

The Perfect Sirtfood Recipes For

All Meals

Now that you know how to eat during the first two phases of the diet, it's time to start learning about the actual meals you should eat. This chapter will focus on a carnivore diet, and give you recipes for breakfast, lunch, and dinner, that are all based on sirtuin-boosting foods. Keep in mind that these recipes are highly adjustable and that you can substitute ingredients for other foods you like better.

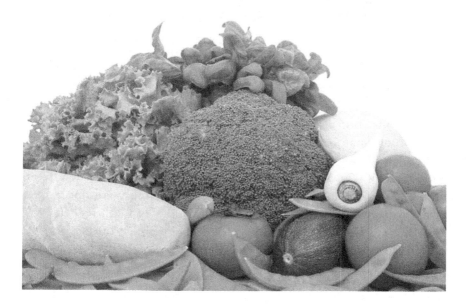

Breakfast

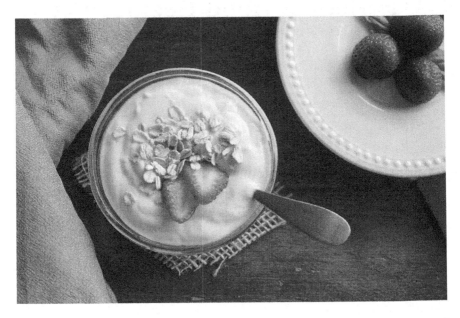

Breakfast is thought to be the most important meal of the day. Ideally, your breakfast should include enough carbs and fiber to supply enough energy to jump-start your morning, but not cause fatigue or drowsiness. The following breakfast recipes are based on sirtuin-boosting foods, but also designed to be delicious and easy to make. Keep in mind that each of these recipes totals up to 350 calories. Depending on your dietary preferences, you might decide to boost your breakfast if you're hungriest in the morning, or slim it down if you don't like eating a lot as soon as you get up. Flexibility is important if you want to stay within a 1,500-calorie daily limit, but still feel full and energized. Here are a couple of ideas for your breakfast during phase 2 of the Sirtfood diet:

Sirt Cereal

Ingredients:

- Buckwheat, 1 oz flakes, and 0.5 oz puffs
- Coconut, either desiccated or flakes, 1.5 oz
- Chopped walnuts, 1.5 0z
- Medjool dates, 1.5 oz
- Chopped strawberries, 3.5 oz
- Cocoa nibs 0.5 oz
- Skim milk, almond/coconut milk or Greek yogurt, plain, 3.5 oz

Instructions:

Soak the dry ingredients in yogurt or milk and top with chopped strawberries. This meal is simple, delicious, and satiating. If you won't be eating right away, serve the yogurt and strawberries last.

Lemony Mint Pancakes With Yogurt Sauce

Ingredients:

Yogurt Sauce

- Juice and peel from one lemon
- Greek yogurt, 1 cup
- A pinch of ground turmeric
- 1 minced garlic clove
- A handful of minced parsley leaves

Pancakes

- 3 large eggs
- 1 cup of finely chopped kale
- Milk, 2 tbsp

- Buckwheat flour, 1 cup
- 1 ½ tsp of ground cumin
- Ground turmeric, to tsp
- Coriander, ground, 1 tsp
- Ground bird's eye chili pepper, ½ tsp
- Garlic powder, ½ tsp
- Whole-wheat flour, 1 cup
- Extra virgin olive oil, 4 tsp

Instructions:

1. Start by making your yogurt sauce. Mix in the ingredients and cool in your freezer until you're ready to serve the dish.
2. Next, make your pancakes. Combine the ingredients and blend together until you get a homogenous batter.
3. Fry 1 tbsp of extra virgin olive oil on medium heat, turning the pancakes to the other side after 2-3 minutes. The batter and oil should suffice for four pancakes.

Chocolate Granola

For this breakfast, you'll be making chocolate granola with maple syrup.

Ingredients:

- Oats, organic, 5 oz
- Walnuts, chopped, 1.7 oz
- Butter, 0.7 oz
- Maple syrup, 2 tbsp
- Chocolate chips (70% cocoa), 2 oz
- Brown sugar, 1 tbsp
- Olive oil, 3 tbsp

Instructions:

1. Preheat your oven to 160 °C. While your oven is heating up, prepare your baking tray.
2. Mix the walnuts into a bowl. Pull out a non-stick pan and heat butter and olive oil with the maple syrup and brown sugar. Once the syrup and sugar have dissolved, top the oat and nut mix and stir until all the dry ingredients are coated.
3. Distribute and spread the granola onto your tray and bake for 20 minutes. When the granola cools down, break it up and mix in with chocolate chips. You can store them in a jar for around two weeks.

Buckwheat With Nuts and Coconut

Ingredients:

- Soy, coconut, or Greek yogurt, 100 g
- Walnuts, chopped, 0. 5 oz
- Buckwheat flakes, ½ cup
- Buckwheat puffs, ⅓ cup
- Coconut flakes or dried coconut, 0. 5 oz
- Chopped Medjool dates, 1.5 oz
- Cocoa nibs, 1.4 oz
- Chopped strawberries, 1 cup

Instructions:

Mix all ingredients and enjoy! If you want to have this mixture ready beforehand, you can mix the dry ingredients and store them in a container. Add yogurt only when you're about to serve.

Pancakes With Blueberries, Banana and Apples

Ingredients:

For Pancakes

- Six bananas
- Blueberries, ¼ cup
- Six eggs
- Rolled oats, 1 ½ cup
- A pinch of salt
- Baking powder, 2 tsp
- For the applesauce
- Two apples
- Two pitted dates
- Lemon juice, 1 tbsp
- A pinch of cinnamon powder
- A pinch of salt

For Turmeric Topping

- Coconut milk, 3 cup
- Ginger root, 1 small piece
- Raw honey, 1 tsp
- Turmeric powder, 1 tsp

Instructions:

1. Start by making your pancakes. First, make the oat flower by pulling the rolled oats in your blender for a minute. Add the remaining ingredients for the batter and blend for two minutes until you've formed a smooth batter. Pour the batter into a bowl and mix in blueberries, making sure that they are evenly distributed across the mixture.

2. Leave to sit for another 10 minutes until the baking powder is activated. Bake on medium on a thin layer of butter or coconut oil. To fry the pancakes evenly, distribute a couple of batter spoons across the pan, wait until it turns golden color, and flip to the other side.

3. Once your pancakes are done, start making the sauce. This step should be simple, and it consists of putting all the ingredients for the sauce into a blender and blending until the mixture is uniform.

4. Now, onto the turmeric topping. Pop all the ingredients into a blender, and then transfer into a small pot and heat on low temperature. The ingredients should melt together to form a syrup-like consistency, but not boil to avoid destroying the nutrients.

Sirtfood Smoothie

Ingredients:

- Berries of your choosing, 2 cup
- 1 ripe banana
- Greek yogurt, 2 tbsp
- Skim milk, 200 ml

Instructions:

Blend all the ingredients together and enjoy!

Sirtfood Melon Smoothie

Ingredients:

- 1 cucumber, peeled and chopped

- Finely chopped spinach leaves, 1 cup
- 1 apple, chopped
- Chia seeds, 1 tbsp
- Red grapes, 1 cup
- Cantaloupe melon, chopped, 1 cup

Instructions:

Blend all the ingredients together and enjoy!

Salads

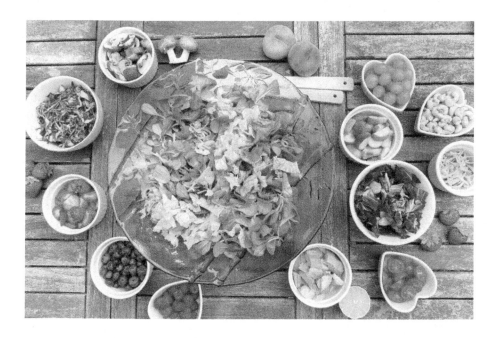

Buckwheat Noodles

Ingredients:

- Shrimps, deveined and shelled, 1 ½ cup
- Extra virgin olive oil, 2 tsp
- Buckwheat noodles, 1 cup
- Soy sauce or tamari (gluten-free), 2 tsp
- 1 chopped garlic clove
- 1 chopped fresh ginger
- 1 freshly chopped bird's eye chili
- Chicken stock, 100 ml
- Sliced red onions, ½ cup
- Chopped kale, ½ cup

- Sliced and trimmed celery, ½ cup
- Celery leaves or lovage, 1 tsp
- Chopped green beans, 1 cup

Instructions:

Cook shrimps with 1 tsp of soy sauce or tamari and 1 tsp of olive oil for a couple of minutes on high heat. Pour the prawns out of the pan and wipe down oil residue with kitchen paper. Cook buckwheat noodles for up to eight minutes, drain and leave on the side to cool off. As your noodles cool down, fry the remaining ingredients (kale, beans, celery, ginger, red onion, chili, and garlic) up to three minutes. Add the stock to the mix and simmer for a couple more minutes. The vegetables should be cooked but still fresh-looking and crunchy. Finally, add the buckwheat noodles, celery, and prawns to the pan, boil briefly, and you're done!

Buckwheat and Strawberries Salad

Ingredients:

- Buckwheat, ½ cup
- Red Onion, ½ cup
- Tomato, 1 cup
- Avocado, 1 cup
- Strawberries, 1 cup
- Parsley, 3 tbsp
- Rocket, 3 tbsp
- Pitted Medjool Dates, ¼ cup
- ½ lemon, juiced
- Capers, 1 tbsp
- Turmeric, ground, 1 tbsp
- Olive Oil, 1 tbsp

Instructions:

To start off with this recipe, check the buckwheat package instructions to cook with turmeric. While your buckwheat cools off, chop parsley, capers, dates, avocado, tomatoes, and the red onion, and mix in with the buckwheat. Top with sliced strawberries, lemon juice, and extra virgin olive oil. Layer the rocket on your plate and top with the mix.

Sirtfood Vegetable Salad

Ingredients:

- 1 finely chopped apple
- Chopped celery, 200 g
- One roughly chopped red onion
- Roughly chopped walnuts, ½ cup
- 1 chopped chicory head
- Chopped parsley, 10 g
- Arugula, 1 tbsp
- Roughly chopped celery leaves,
- Extra virgin olive oil, 1 tbsp
- Lemon juice, ½ tbsp
- Mustard, 1 tsp

Instructions:

Mix the celery, arugula, onion, walnuts, and parsley in a bowl and toss together. Mix the extra virgin olive oil, lemon juice, and mustard. Drizzle over the salad and enjoy!

Arugula Side-Salad

Ingredients:

- Arugula, 2 ½ cups

- Smoked salmon, sliced, 1 ⅕ oz
- Low-fat ricotta, 1 cup
- Sliced celery with leaves, ½ cup
- 1 sliced red onion
- Chopped walnuts, 1 tbsp
- Capers, 1 tbsp
- 1 chopped date
- Extra virgin olive oil, 1 tbsp

Instructions:

Mix all ingredients together in a bowl and enjoy!

Apple and Lime Sirtfood Salad

Ingredients:
- 1 green apple
- 6 chopped walnuts
- Chopped celery, 1 cup
- Finely chopped ginger, 1 tbsp
- Chopped Kale, 1 cup
- Lime juice, 1 tbsp
- Parsley, 1 tbsp
- Arugula, 1 cup
- A pinch of salt
- A pinch of pepper
- Extra virgin olive oil, 1 tbsp

Instructions:

Mix all of the ingredients together and enjoy!

Quick Sirtfood Chicken Salad

Ingredients:

- Diced chicken breasts, 5 oz
- Greek yogurt, 1 cup
- Lime juice, 1 tbsp
- Ground turmeric, 1 tsp
- Chopped coriander, 1 tsp
- Curry powder, ½ tsp
- Chopped walnuts, 1 cup
- 2 finely chopped Medjool dates
- Arugula, 1 cup
- 1 bird's eye chili
- 1 diced red onion

Instructions:

1. Cook chicken breasts until ready per your taste and set aside to cool down.
2. Mix the dry ingredients into a bowl, add the chicken breasts, top with lime juice and extra virgin olive oil.

Meat

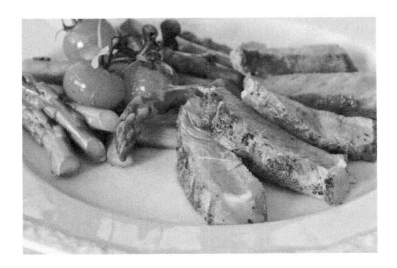

Savory Chicken With Kale and Ricotta Salad

Ingredients:

- Extra virgin olive oil, 1 tbsp
- 1 diced red onion
- 1 finely diced garlic cove
- Juice and zest from ½ lemon
- Diced chicken meat of your choosing, 300 g
- A pinch of salt
- A pinch of pepper

For salad

- Pumpkin seeds, 2 tbsp
- Finely chopped kale, 2 cup
- Ricotta cheese, ½ cup
- Coriander leaves, chopped, ¼ cup

- Parsley Leaves, chopped, ¼ cup

Salad dressing

- Orange juice, 3 tbsp
- 1 finely minced garlic clove
- Extra virgin olive oil, 3 tbsp
- Raw honey, 1 tsp
- Wholegrain mustard, ½ tsp
- A pinch of salt
- A pinch of pepper

Instructions:

1. Start by cooking chicken. Heat the oil over medium-high heat and add the onions. Let the onions sauté up to five minutes. Once the onions turn a golden color, add the chicken and garlic. If you'd like to finish quickly, stir-fry for up to three minutes at medium-high temperature, or lower the temperature and let it slowly simmer for up to fifteen minutes. The latter option will result in soft chicken, while the medium-heat stir fry will produce crunchy meat dices.
2. Next, add the lemon juice, pepper, zest, and turmeric during the last four minutes of cooking.
3. While your chicken is cooking, prepare the kale. While you can blanch the vegetable in boiling water up to two minutes, I'd recommend microwaving with ½ cup of water up to five minutes to preserve nutrients.
4. Remember, kale is edible raw, and cooking only serves to achieve the desired flavor and consistency. You can microwave the kale for as short as two minutes if all you need is for it to soften up, and the full five minutes if you prefer that fully-cooked taste.

5. During the last two minutes of chicken cooking, toss in the pumpkin seeds and stir fry. Remove from heat and set aside.
6. Mix both dishes into a bowl and add ricotta and the remaining fresh herbs. Enjoy!

Sirtfood Chicken Breasts

Ingredients:

- Chicken breasts, 5 oz
- Chopped Kale, 1 cup
- Red Onion, sliced, ½ cup
- Buckwheat, 1 cup
- Fresh ginger, chopped, 1 tsp
- Olive Oil, extra virgin, 1 tbsp
- Turmeric, ground, 2 tsp
- ¼ lemon, juiced

Salsa

- Tomato, chopped, 1 cup
- 1 chopped bird's eye's chili
- Capers, finely chopped, 1 tbsp
- Parsley, finely chopped, 1 tsp
- ¼ lemon, juiced

Instructions:

1. Chop the tomato while making sure not to squish it and preserve the maximum liquid in the process. Add the lemon juice, parsley, capers, and chili. Pop everything into a blender and you're done!
2. Heat your oven to 220 °C. While your oven is heating, marinate the chicken with turmeric, olive oil, and the lemon juice up to

15 minutes. Cook in an ovenproof pan on each side until the chicken turns pale golden. Transfer to the oven and bake for 10 minutes, cover with foil, and cook for another five minutes.

3. While your chicken is baking, steam the kale for five minutes, adding red onions, ginger, and little oil. Mix and fry for up to five minutes. To make the second side dish, cook buckwheat with turmeric according to instructions on the package and serve all together.

Turkey With Sirtfood Vegetables

This recipe is highly adjustable, and it's based on combining turkey as the main dish with healthy side-dishes made of vegetables. It's extremely simple and convenient, as meats go great with any and all Sirt spices and vegetables. With that in mind, feel free to adjust or replace any ingredient in this recipe with an equal amount of the ingredients you prefer or like better.

Ingredients:
- Lean turkey meat, 150 g
- 1 finely chopped garlic clove
- 1 finely chopped red onion
- 1 finely chopped bird's eye chili/replace with chopped red bell paprika or ½ squeezed citrus fruit if you don't like spicy foods
- 1 tsp of finely chopped ginger
- Extra virgin olive oil, 2 tbsp
- Ground turmeric, 1 tbsp
- ½ cup of dried tomatoes
- Parsley, 10 g
- Sage, dried, 1 tsp
- ½ juiced lime or lemon
- Capers, 1 tbsp

Instructions:

1. Chop the cauliflower. Fry with chopped ginger, chili, red onion, and garlic in 1 tbsp olive oil until they're soft. Add cauliflower and turmeric, and cook for a couple of minutes until the cauliflower becomes soft. Once the dish is done, add dried tomatoes and parsley.
2. Coat your turkey in a thin layer of olive oil and sage. Fry for about five minutes, and then add the capers and lime juice to the mix. Add half a cup of water and bring to a boil.

Sirtfood Beef

Ingredients:

- 1 large beef steak
- 1 diced potato
- Extra virgin olive oil, 1 tbsp
- Finely chopped parsley, ½ tbsp
- One sliced red onion
- Sliced kale, 1 cup
- Beef stock, 150 ml
- 1 finely chopped garlic clove
- Red wine, ½ cup
- Tomato sauce, 1 tsp
- 1 tbsp water
- Corn flour, 1 tsp

Instructions:

1. Preheat your oven to 220 °C
2. Boil the potatoes in a saucepan for 4-5 minutes, transfer into the oven and roast for 30-45 with a little bit of olive oil. Turn every ten minutes so that the potatoes are roasted evenly. Pull

out of the oven and add chopped parsley. Fry onions and garlic in a little bit of olive oil and add kale after a minute. Fry another two minutes until it turns soft.

3. Coat the meat in a thin layer of oil and fry on medium heat until it's cooked the way you like it. Remove from the pan add the wine into the remaining oil and leave to bubble. Once the wine is reduced by half and appears thicker, you can pour into the stock and tomato sauce and bring to a boil. Add corn flour paste until you achieve the desired consistency. Serve with the steak and vegetables.

Sirtfood Beans With Beef

Ingredients:

- Kidney beans, 2 small cans
- Lean beef, minced, 400 g
- Buckwheat, 160 g
- 1 finely chopped red onion
- 1 chopped red bell pepper
- Two finely chopped bird's eye chili peppers
- Canned tomatoes, 800 g
- Ground turmeric, 1 tbsp
- Tomato sauce, 1 tbsp
- Cocoa powder, 1 tbsp
- Ground cumin, 1 tbsp
- Extra virgin olive oil, 1 tbsp
- Red wine, 150 ml
- Chopped coriander, ½ tbsp.
- Chopped parsley, ½ tbsp.

Instructions:

- Fry the onions, chili peppers, and garlic for three minutes over medium heat. Throw in the spices and mince for another minute. After that, add the beef and red wine. Bring to a boil and let it bubble until the liquid reduces by a half.
- Add the cocoa powder, tomatoes, tomato sauce, and the red bell pepper. Add more water if needed and let the dish simmer on low medium heat for an hour. Add the remaining chopped herbs before serving.

Chicken and Kale Buckwheat Noodles

This tasty dish will take no more than 30 minutes to prepare, prep time included.

Ingredients:

For noodles

- Finely chopped kale, 2 cup
- Buckwheat noodles, 5 oz
- Shiitake mushrooms (or any other of your choosing), four pieces
- Extra virgin olive oil, 1 tsp
- 1 finely diced red onion
- 1 diced chicken breast
- 1 sliced bird's eye chili
- Soy sauce, 3 tbsp

Salad dressing

- Soy sauce, ¼ cup
- Tamari sauce, 1 tbsp
- Sesame oil, 1 tbsp

- Lemon juice, 1 tbsp

Instructions:

1. Boil or stir-fry chicken for up to 15 minutes.
2. Microwave kale up to three minutes to preserve nutrients.
3. Cook buckwheat noodles and rinse and add kale once they're done.
4. Fry the mushrooms with 1 tsp of olive oil up to three minutes and season with a pinch of salt. Set aside and use the same pan, adding more olive oil, to sauté peppers and chickpeas up to five minutes. Add garlic, water, and tamari sauce, and cook for another three minutes. Add kale with noodles, chicken, and dressing. Mix all together and serve.

Sirtfood Lamb

Ingredients:

- Extra virgin olive oil, 2 tbsp
- Grated ginger, one inch
- 1 sliced red onion.
- 1 tsp of bird's eye
- Cumin seeds, 2 tsp
- 1 cinnamon stick
- Lamb, 800 g
- Garlic cloves, crushed, 3 pieces
- A pinch of salt
- Chopped Medjool dates, 1 cup
- Chickpeas, 400 g
- Coriander, 2 tbsp
- Buckwheat

Instructions:

1. Start by preheating your oven to 140 °C. Sauté sliced onion with 2 tbsp of extra virgin olive oil for five minutes while keeping the lid on. The onions should turn soft but not brown.

2. Add turmeric, cumin, ginger, garlic, and chili and stir fry for another minute.

3. Add the chunks of lamb, season with salt and let, and let boil. Add a glass of water.

4. After the mixture has boiled, roast in the oven for one hour and 15 minutes. Add the chickpeas half an hour before the dish is finished.

5. Add chopped coriander and serve with buckwheat after the meal is done.

Fish

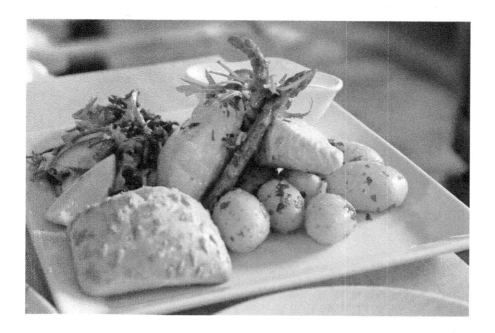

Savory Sirtfood Salmon

Ingredients:

- Salmon, 5 oz
- Lemon juice, 1 tbsp
- Ground turmeric, 1 tsp
- Extra virgin olive oil, 2 tbsp
- 1 chopped red onion
- 1 finely chopped garlic clove
- 1 finely chopped bird's eye chili
- Quinoa, 2 oz
- Finely chopped ginger, fresh, 1 tsp
- Celery, chopped, 1 cup

- Parsley, chopped, 1 tbsp
- Tomato, diced, 4.5 oz
- Vegetable stock, 100 ml

Instructions:

Preheat your oven to 200 °C. Fry the celery, chili, garlic, onion, and ginger on olive oil up to three minutes. Add quinoa, tomatoes, and the chicken stock and let simmer for another ten minutes.

Layer olive oil, lemon juice, and turmeric on top of the salmon and bake for ten minutes. Add parsley and celery before serving.

Fish With Mango and Turmeric

Ingredients:
- A fresh 1 ¼ lbs piece of fish of your choosing
- ½ cup of coconut oil
- A pinch of sea salt
- 1 tbsp of high-quality red wine
- ¼ cup olive oil
- ½ tbsp minced ginger
- Scallion, 2 cup
- Dill, 2 cup
- 1 ripe mango
- 1 squeezed lemon
- 1 garlic clove
- Dry red pepper, 1 tsp
- Fresh cilantro
- Walnuts

Instructions:
1. Marinate the fish and leave overnight

2. Blend the ingredients for mango dipping sauce
3. Fry the fish in 2 tbsp in coconut oil on medium heat and add a pinch of salt after five minutes. Turn to the other side and fry for another couple of minutes. Keep the remaining oil in the pan. Add scallions and dill and turn off the heat. Heat for about 15 seconds and season with a pinch of salt.
4. Top the fish with the infused oil, dill, and scallion and serve with the mango sauce, nuts, lime, and cilantro.

Sirtfood Shrimp Noodles

Ingredients:
- Shrimps, deveined ⅓ lb
- Soy sauce, 2 tsp
- Extra virgin olive oil, 2 tsp
- Buckwheat noodles, 3oz
- 2 finely chopped garlic cloves
- 1 bird's eye chili, finely chopped
- Chopped fresh ginger, 1 tsp
- Chopped red onion, ¼
- Chopped celery with eaves, ½ cup
- Chopped green beans, ½ cup
- Chopped kale, 1 cup
- Chicken stock, ½ cup

Instructions:
- Cook the shrimps in 1 tsp of the soy sauce and one tsp of the oil up to three minutes on high heat.
- Cook buckwheat noodles for up to eight minutes and drain.
- Fry the remaining ingredients in a pan on medium heat for up to three minutes. Add the chicken stock, bring to a boil, and

cook until the veggies are cooked, but still look fresh. Add the shrimps and noodles, bring to a boil, and you're done!

Sirtfood Miso Salmon

Ingredients:

- Miso, ½ cup
- Organic red wine, 1 tbsp
- Extra virgin olive oil, 1 tbsp
- Salmon, 7 oz
- 1 sliced red onion
- Celery, sliced, 1 cup
- 2 finely chopped garlic cloves
- 1 finely chopped bird's eye chili
- Ground turmeric, 1 tsp
- Freshly chopped ginger, 1 tsp
- Green beans, 1 cup
- Kale, finely chopped, 1 cup
- Sesame seeds. 1 tsp
- Soy sauce, 1 tbsp
- Buckwheat, 2 tbsp

Instructions:

1. Marinate the salmon in the mix of red wine, 1 tsp of extra virgin olive oil, and miso for 30 minutes. Preheat your oven to 420 °F and bake the fish for ten minutes.
2. Fry the onions, chili, garlic, green beans, ginger, kale, and celery for a few minutes until it's cooked. Insert the soy sauce, parsley, and sesame seeds.
3. Cook buckwheat per instructions and mix in with the stir-fry. Enjoy!

Sirtfood Salmon With Kale Salad

Ingredients:

- Salmon, 4 oz
- 2 sliced red onions
- Parsley, chopped, 1 oz
- Cucumber, 2 oz
- 2 sliced radishes
- Spinach, ½ cup
- Salad leaves, ½ cup

Salad dressing

- Raw honey, 1 tsp
- Greek yogurt, 1 tbsp
- Lemon juice, 1 tbsp
- Chopped mint leaves, 2 tbsp
- A pinch of salt
- A pinch of pepper

Instructions:

1. Preheat your oven to 200 °C. Bake the salmon for up to 18 minutes and set aside. Mix in the ingredients for dressing and leave to sit between five and ten minutes.
2. Serve the salad with spinach and top with parsley, onions, cucumber, and radishes.

Sirtfood Shrimps With Buckwheat Noodles

Ingredients:

- Shrimps (or a piece of fish of your choosing), 4 oz
- Tamari, 2 tbsp

- Extra virgin olive oil, 2 tbsp
- Buckwheat noodles, 75 g
- 1 finely chopped bird's eye chili
- 1 finely chopped garlic clove
- Fresh ginger, chopped, 1 tsp
- 1 sliced red onion
- Sliced red celery, ½ cup
- Chopped green beans, 1 cup
- Chopped kale, 1 cup
- Chicken stock, 1 cup
- Celery, 1 tsp

Instructions:

1. Cook the shrimps for three minutes on high heat and with 1 tsp of tamari and 1 tsp of extra virgin olive oil. Set aside.
2. Cook the noodles for up to eight minutes and set aside.
3. Fry kale, beans, celery, and onion, ginger, chili, and garlic in oil for up to three minutes. Add vegetable stock and simmer for two minutes.
4. Mix all together, bring to a boil, and serve.

Sirtfood Shellfish Salad

Ingredients:

- Tomato sauce, 1 tsp
- Cloves, ¼ tsp
- Coriander, chopped, 1 tbsp
- Parsley, chopped, 1 tbsp
- Lemon juice, 1 tbsp (½ of a lemon)
- Kale, chopped, 1 cup
- Spinach, chopped, 1 cup

- Sea fruit of your choosing (shrimps, prawns, or clamps), 1 cup
- Chopped firm tofu, 1 thick slice (approx. 4 oz)
- Buckwheat noodles, 1 cup
- Pecan nuts, ½ cup
- Chopped ginger, ½ cup
- Miso paste, 1 tbsp
- Carrots, ½ cup
- Chicken stock, 100 ml

Instructions:

Simmer tomato sauce with lemon juice, chicken stock, coriander, parsley, and shrimps/cloves/clams for 10 minutes on medium heat. Add the remaining ingredients without the ginger and miso, and stir-fry until the shellfish is cooked through. Add the remaining seasonings, and you're done!

Snacks

Sirtfood Pizza

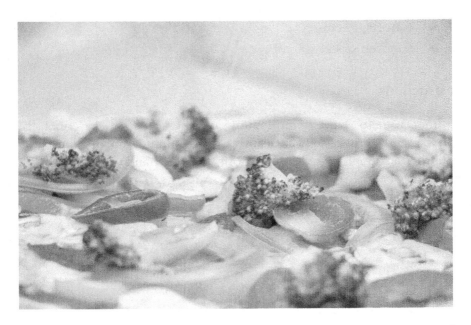

Sirtfood Pizzas are delicious and satiating, aside from being low-carb, low-calorie, and nutrient-rich. While you don't have to bake entirely Sirtfood pizzas to follow this diet plan, and instead you can just add individual Sirt foods to your favorite pizza, these recipes will fit into your 1,000-1,500 daily calorie limit. Here's how to bake two small Sirtfood pizzas:

Ingredients:

Base

- Flour, 14 oz (½ buckwheat flour, ½ rice or white flour)
- Water, 3 cup
- 1 bag of dried yeast

- 1 tbsp of extra virgin olive oil
- 1 tsp of brown sugar

Sauce

- 14 oz of chopped tomatoes, fresh or canned
- ½ chopped red onion
- 1 chopped garlic clove
- 2 tbsp of red wine
- 1 tsp of extra virgin olive oil
- Dried oregano, 1 tsp
- Basil leaves, 1 tsp

Toppings

- Grilled eggplant, red onion, arugula
- Cherry tomato, chili flakes, cottage cheese or mozzarella
- Olives, cooked chicken
- Kale (fresh and steamed), chorizo, mushrooms, red onions

Instructions:

1. Start off by making the dough. First, dissolve the yeast in water and add sugar. Leave up to 15 minutes covered in clingfilm.
2. Next, slowly pour the flour into the bowl. Pay attention not to create clumps as you pour the flour into the yeast.
3. Add the extra virgin olive oil and start mixing the dough. Proceed to knead until the mix is smooth, consistent, and thick.
4. Leave the dough to rise up to 60 minutes in an oiled bowl, after you've covered it with a damp cloth or a tea towel. You'll know the dough has risen enough when it doubles in size.
5. While your dough rises, start making your sauce. Start by frying chopped garlic and onion in a small dose of olive oil. Once the onion softens, pour in the wine and add dried oregano. Proceed cooking until the mixture reduces by half.

6. Add chopped tomatoes, stir, and pour the sugar into the sauce. Proceed cooking for another 30 minutes. Wait until your dough rises and knead for a couple more minutes to remove the air bubbles. Heat your oven to 220 °C. Dust your kitchen counter with flour, split the dough into halves, and roll out the pieces until you like their thickness. Transfer onto the baking tray or the pizza stone.

7. Now layer the tomato sauce over the dough and leave a small gap along the edges. Add the toppings you like, and in quantities you prefer. However, make sure to add any heat sensitive ingredients, like arugula or chili, after you've baked the pizza. Leave for another 15 minutes for the dough to start rising again. Bake for up to 12 minutes. Once your pizza is out of the oven, add fresh herbs and toppings of your choosing.

Great job! You now know which meals to cook during your Sirtfood diet calorie restriction. Rest assured that these recipes will help you feel full and energized throughout the entire day. Here are some general tips and tricks for more convenient Sirtfood cooking:

- **Be practical.** Most of the recipes given in this chapter won't take longer than 30-45 minutes to make. However, you can make the process even faster and easier by pre-making meals the day or night before, or cooking larger amounts of meat and vegetables and storing your meals in the fridge.

- **Invest in quality pots.** Quality cooking supplies guarantee that you'll be able to stir-fry without using a lot of oil. The majority of recipes given in this chapter are easy to cook with no more than 2 tbsp of extra virgin olive oil. But, without the right dishes, it could happen that your foods start to stick to the bottom of the pan. In this case, instead of adding more oil, simply pour a little bit of water.

- **Substitutes.** Don't like some of the ingredients provided in these recipes? Or, you find some of them difficult to find or expensive to purchase? Don't worry! Each of these meals can be adjusted according to your taste. Here are a couple of substitutes that you can use for some of the ingredients:

- ○ **Meat**. You can substitute different types of meat for an equal amount of any other meat you like. You can also substitute meat with mushrooms, potatoes, eggs, and beans.

- ○ **Fruit**. If you don't want to use avocados, you can replace them with bananas or melons. Melons have a similar consistency, and while they don't taste the same as avocados, they won't significantly alter a dish.

- ○ **Buckwheat**. As you may have noticed, buckwheat is heavily featured in the majority of recipes. If you don't want to eat that much of it, you can switch it with an equal amount of quinoa, kale, spinach, or beans. Keep in mind that doing so will affect the steps in cooking, and may affect preparation time. If you're not using leafy greens to substitute buckwheat, but you're using beans or legumes instead, it would be the best to cook the substitutes beforehand, and add them to other dishes as they're being cooked.

Chapter 5:

Vegetarian Sirtfood Recipes

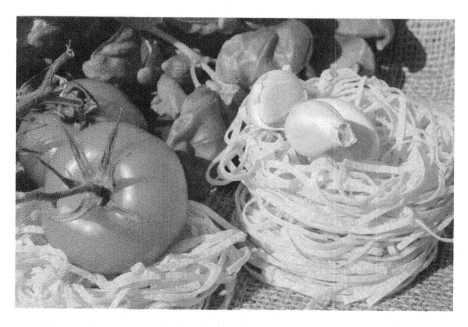

You can follow the Sirtfood diet even if you're a vegetarian or a vegan. The 20 superfoods and the diet principles that aim to trigger your 'skinny' gene don't include any animal ingredients, meaning that you can have all the Sirt foods you want and in abundant amounts. Aside from that, this diet doesn't exclude any plant-based foods from your daily meal plan, meaning that you most likely won't have to give up your favorite go-to meals throughout the diet.

However, due to the calorie restrictions in the first two phases of the diet, you should give your nutrition some extra attention and even use supplements if needed to make sure you're covered with the essential nutrients. Compared to the carnivore diet, calorie restriction during the first two weeks can feel extra hard, because you might be deprived of the nutrients otherwise found in meat and dairy, like protein. To secure healthy nutrition during the diet, you should supplement iodine, calcium, omega-3 fatty acids, and vitamin B12.

Sirt foods are compatible with any other diet approach you might be following, and don't require you to eliminate any food groups. The only restrictive element of the diet revolves around calories. During the first week, even as a vegetarian, your calorie count will total 1,000 calories, and you should aim for 1,500 calories during your second week. With this in mind, you should still aim to design your meals so that 50% of your serving consists of healthy, organic carbs, 25% fiber (fruits and vegetables), and 25% protein (meats or protein-dense plants). Taking this into consideration, you should aim to have 750 calories-worth of carbs, 350 calories from fiber, and 350 calories from protein-based foods. While there's no secure way to ensure your proportions are accurate, getting as close to these numbers will give your body all the nutrition it needs to function properly, despite the calorie restriction.

Research showed that even people with chronic illnesses felt well and improved not only their weight but also blood sugar and blood pressure when their diet was balanced. Numerous studies recorded similar results even when participants with obesity were put on highly restrictive, 1000-calorie daily diets, and even when they fasted for longer periods. This only goes to show that calorie restriction doesn't have to be difficult if you balance out your meals.

Keeping in mind that healthy carbs do provide an immediate energy source for you to feel good while your body burns fat, you can turn to starchy Sirt foods (soy, onions, kale, and buckwheat) and make them as abundant in your portions as possible while sticking to the maximum daily intake recommendations.

Aside from vegan and vegetarian, the Sirtfood diet is also compatible with gluten-free, low-carb, paleo, ketogenic, and intermittent fasting diet. If your diet is low-carb, and you feel like you're not having enough fruits and vegetables, which is all too common for the majority of people who don't have the time to study and plan their diets, the Sirtfood diet can be a really simple way to enhance your diet without additional calories. With a simple list of foods needed to reap the health benefits, you won't have a problem incorporating these foods without compromising your diet concept.

Breakfast

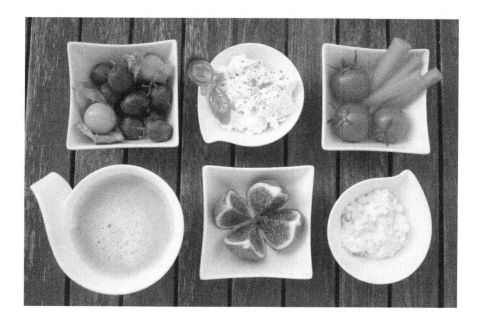

Eggs and Sirtfood Vegetables

Ingredients:

- 1 eggs
- Kale, chopped, 1 cup
- Chopped parsley, 1 tbsp
- Chopped red onion, ½ cup
- Extra virgin olive oil, 1 tsp

- 1 finely chopped garlic clove
- Finely chopped celery, ½ cup
- 1 finely chopped paprika or bird's eye chili
- Ground turmeric, 1 tsp
- Ground cumin, 1 tsp
- Paprika, 1 tsp
- 1 14 oz can of sliced tomatoes

Instructions:

Fry the chili, spices, garlic, onion, and celery for a minute or two in olive oil, add the tomato sauce and let it simmer for 20 minutes. Pop the kale into the pan and cook for another five minutes, adding more water as needed. Lastly, add the parsley. Break the eggs and stir into the sauce, or boil them and serve next to the sauce.

Vegetarian Sirtfood Omelet

Ingredients:

- 2 eggs
- Kale, chopped, ½ cup
- Ground turmeric, 1 tsp
- Ginger, finely chopped, 1 tsp
- 1 sliced bird's eye chili
- Extra virgin olive oil, 1 tsp

Instructions:

Mix all ingredients together. Optionally, you can blend for a minute if you prefer a homogenous-looking omelet. Fry in olive oil. First, layer the eggs across the frying pan and wait for the edges to turn dry and golden. Flip and fry on the other side.

Sirtfood Fruit Yogurt

Ingredients:

- Strawberries, chopped, 1 cup
- Raspberries, 1 cup
- Greek yogurt, 2 cup
- Chia seeds, 1 tbsp

Instructions:

Blend the berries with Greek yogurt and chia seeds and enjoy!

Buckwheat Apple Pancakes

This recipe will give your four quick, healthy, and delicious pancakes.

Ingredients:

- Two eggs
- Buckwheat flour, 2 cup
- Sugar, 2 tbsp
- A pinch of salt
- Two chopped, peeled apples
- Skim milk, 3 cup
- Olive oil, 2 tsp
- Baking powder, 1 tsp

Instructions:

1. Cook apples in a small amount of water, up to ½ cup and let boil up to two minutes. Blend to create a sauce.
2. Now, start making pancakes. Mix baking powder, the flour, and sugar into a bowl. Add milk and mix until the texture is even and smooth. Mix in both eggs.

3. Fry ¼ of the batter on ½ tsp of olive oil on medium high heat. Repeat four times, until you fry all of the batter.

Lunch

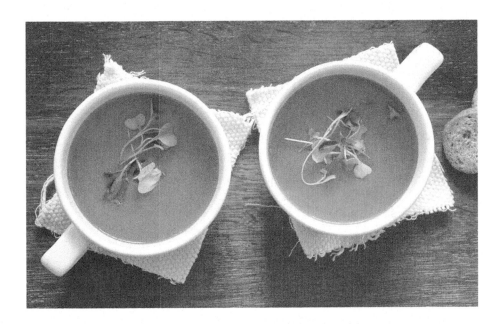

Sirtfood Lentils

Ingredients:

- 1 cup chopped cherry tomatoes
- Extra virgin olive oil, 2 tsp
- 1 finely chopped red onion
- 1 finely chopped garlic clove
- Celery, thin-sliced, ½ cup
- Carrots, diced, ½ cup
- Paprika or bird's eye chili, 1 tsp

- Thyme, dry or fresh, 1 tsp
- Parsley, 1 tbsp
- Arugula, 20 g
- Chopped kale, 1 cup
- Lentils, 1 cup
- Vegetable stock, 220 ml

Instructions:

1. Preheat your oven to 120 °C
2. Roast the tomatoes for 30 minutes
3. Stir-fry paprika/bird-eye chili, garlic, red onion, carrot, and celery on 1 tsp olive oil. Once the vegetables have softened, add paprika and thyme. Add vegetable stock. Cook for another minute or two. Rinse your lentils and add to the pan until the mixture boils. Reduce the heat and simmer lightly for another 20 minutes. Stir regularly and add water if you feel like the mix is becoming too dry.
4. Add kale to the mix, wait another 10 minutes, and stir in roasted tomatoes and parsley. Top with fresh arugula and drizzle with lemon juice and olive oil.

Eggs With Zucchini and Onions

Ingredients:

- 4 eggs
- Olive oil, 1 tsp
- 1 finely chopped onion
- 1 red chili pepper, finely chopped
- 1 finely chopped garlic clove
- 1 finely chopped zucchini
- Tomato sauce, 1 tbsp

- A pinch of salt
- A pinch of Bird's eye chili powder
- A pinch of ground cumin
- Chopped tomatoes, 14 oz
- Canned quinoa, 14 oz
- Chopped parsley, ⅓ oz

Instructions:

1. Fry onions and peppers up to five minutes in a thin layer of oil in a saucepan on low temperature. Add the zucchini and garlic, bring to a boil, and then add tomato sauce, salt, and spices. Stir and add quinoa and chopped tomatoes. Increase the heat to medium-high and let simmer for 30 minutes until the sauce reduces by a third.
2. Remove from the stove, add chopped parsley, and preheat your oven to 200 °C. Add the eggs to the dish without stirring, cover with foil, and bake up to 15 minutes.

Tomato and Buckwheat Salad

Ingredients:

- Buckwheat noodles, 12 cup
- Arugula, 1 cup
- Basil leaves, 2 pieces
- 1 large chopped tomato
- Grilled tofu, 1 slice, chopped
- Olives, 12 cups
- Walnuts, ½ cup
- Extra virgin olive oil, 1 tbsp
- Lemon juice, 1 tbsp

Instructions:

Cook buckwheat noodles per instructions on the packaging. Mix the remaining ingredients together to make a salad. Add drained buckwheat noodles and drizzle with the olive oil and the lemon juice.

Grilled Mushroom and Tofu Summer Salad

Ingredients:
- Black olives, ½ cup
- 1 chopped tomato
- 1 chopped Bird's eye chili pepper
- Sliced red onion, ½
- 1 sliced cucumber
- Grilled tofu, cubed, 1 cup
- Mushrooms of your choosing, 2 cup
- Parsley, 1 tsp
- Basil, 1 tsp
- Ginger (optional), 1 tsp

Instructions:

1. Grill mushrooms and tofu on a thin layer of olive oil for up to five minutes. Mushrooms can, but don't have to be fully fried, depending on the type.
2. Next, mix in the remaining vegetables and add the freshly fried mushrooms with tofu. Mix all together, add parsley, basil, and ginger, and drizzle with lemon juice and olive oil.

Sirtfood Tofu Sesame Salad

Ingredients:

- Sesame seeds, 1 tbsp
- 1 sliced cucumber
- Kale, chopped, 1 cup
- Arugula, 1 cup
- 1 fine sliced red onion
- Chopped parsley, ¼ cup
- Grilled tofu, diced, 2 cups
- Extra virgin olive oil, 2 tbsp
- Lime juice, 2 tbsp
- Soy sauce, 2 tbsp
- Raw honey, 1 tsp

Instructions:

1. First, start by roasting sesame seeds for up to two minutes. Set aside to cool. If you've bought raw tofu, grill briefly on a thin layer of olive oil. Leave the remaining oil for salad dressing.
2. Mix vegetables and spices into a bowl. Toss in the chopped grilled tofu and sesame seeds, and mix to distribute evenly throughout the salad. To finish off, drizzle with lime juice and olive oil.

Sweet Arugula and Salmon Salad

Ingredients:

- Arugula, ½ cup
- Chicory leaves, ½ cup
- Lentils, 1 cup
- 1 sliced red onion

- Sliced avocado, 80 g
- Sliced celery, ½ cup
- Chopped walnuts, 1 tbsp
- 1 pitted, chopped, Medjool date
- Extra virgin olive oil, 1 tbsp
- Lime juice, 1 tbsp
- Chopped parsley, 1 tbsp
- Celery leaves, chopped, 1 tbsp

Instructions:

Mix all ingredients into a bowl. Drizzle with lime juice and olive oil, spread on a large plate, and enjoy!

Dinner

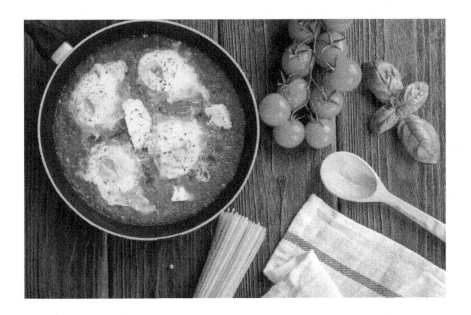

Sirtfood Curry

Ingredients:

- Skim milk
- Quinoa, 2 cup
- Chickpeas, 4 cup
- Potatoes, 14 oz
- Spinach, 1 ½ cup
- Tomato sauce, 1 tbsp
- 3 crushed garlic cloves
- Ground ginger, 1 tsp
- Ground turmeric, 3 tsp
- Ground coriander, 1 tsp
- Bird's eye chili powder, 1 tsp

- A pinch of salt
- A pinch of pepper

Instructions:

Cook the potatoes for up to 30 minutes and drain. Move to a large pan and add all the ingredients except quinoa and bring to a boil. Once the mixture has boiled, add the quinoa and chickpeas, and up to 1 ½ cup of water if needed. Lower the heat and let simmer for 30 minutes while mixing regularly.

Buckwheat Noodles With Tomato and Shrimp

Ingredients:

- Raw shrimps, 2 cup
- Buckwheat noodles, 1 cup
- Extra virgin olive oil, 1 tbsp
- One finely chopped garlic clove
- One finely chopped red onion
- Finely chopped celery, ¼ of a cup
- One finally chopped bird's eye chili
- Organic red wine, 2 tbsp
- Tomato sauce, 4 cup
- Chopped parsley, 1 tbsp

Instructions:

Fry the garlic, onions, chili and celery in extra virgin olive oil for two minutes over medium heat. Add the red wine and tomato sauce and cook for another 30 minutes. Add water if needed. Prepare the buckwheat noodles while the sauce is cooking. Add pasta to the sauce when cooked. And the shrimps and cook for another four minutes. When the dish is cooked, add chopped parsley and serve.

Onion Mushroom Salsa

Ingredients:

- Mushrooms, 1 ⅕ cups
- Ground turmeric, 2 tsp
- Lime juice, 1 tbsp
- Chopped Kale, 1 cup
- 1 sliced red onion
- Arugula, 1 cup
- Fresh ginger, chopped, 1 tsp

Instructions:

Fry the mushrooms on a thin layer of extra virgin olive oil for up to five minutes, while stirring and making sure they're cooking evenly. As you fry, sprinkle turmeric over the mushrooms. Add kale half-way through, letting it soften only lightly. Prepare a plate and lay out fresh arugula.

Mix the remaining ingredients together to make a salsa. If you'd like a more sauce-like consistency, you can blend the vegetables, spices, and the remaining oil. Serve one dish next to another and enjoy!

Arugula With Smoked Salmon

Ingredients:

- Smoked salmon, sliced, 4 oz
- Chopped arugula, 1 cup
- Chopped parsley, 1 tsp
- 2 eggs
- Extra virgin olive oil

Instructions:

Crack and mix the eggs. Roll slices of smoked salmon gently, and sprinkle with chopped parsley. Fry on one tablespoon of extra virgin olive oil briefly, up to two minutes on each side. Serve next to arugula and enjoy!

Sirtfood Striped Bass Fillet

Ingredients:

- Extra virgin olive oil, 2 tbsp
- Striped bass fillet, skinless, 7 oz
- 1 sliced red onion
- 1 finely chopped garlic clove
- 1 finely chopped red bell paprika
- Sliced celery, ½ cup
- Green beans, 1 cup
- Chopped kale, 1 cup
- Parsley, chopped, 1 tsp
- Soy sauce, 1 tbsp
- Ground turmeric, 1 tsp

Instructions:

1. Rub the bass with olive oil and bake for 10 minutes at 220 °C.
2. Fry the remaining ingredients together (without say sauce and parsley) in a pan with remaining extra virgin olive oil. Once the green beans and kale have cooked through, add some water. Finish by adding soy sauce and parsley. Serve with the fish.

In this chapter, you learned how to eat Sirt Foods on a vegetarian diet. While the majority of ingredients for these meals are simple, easy, and affordable, it could happen that you can't find some of them in stores, or simply don't like a few of the original choices. For this reason, you can substitute ingredients as you like. The most important thing to keep in mind is that your meals should mainly consist of Sirtfoods. If you want to diversify your menu, you can use some of the recipes from the previous chapters. You can substitute meats for eggs, beans, and legumes of your choosing. Here are some general tips for making these recipes:

- Stick to whole foods. Store-bought fruits and vegetables not only have less nutritional value, but also lack freshness, crunchiness, and consistency when cooked. It could happen that a pack of store-bought veggies has significantly less flavor than if you used organic options.

- Buy fresh foods. Frozen goods can contain a lot of water, and lose in volume once cooked. This can significantly impact the taste of your meals. If you're cooking with frozen foods, make sure to wait until they thaw, drain them to remove excess water, add more of the same ingredient if it has appeared to have lost some of its mass, and double-check the quantities before cooking.

- Be careful with fish and seafood. Food poisoning from fish and seafood is quite common, and equally unpleasant to experience. Always check the expiration dates on the packaging! The same can be said for making fish, shrimps, prawns, or clams. All of these, particularly if bought frozen, may lose some of their freshness once they thaw. For this reason, make sure to clean and drain the foods before cooking. If you're using frozen instead of fresh, you might find that the foods don't have as intense of a taste as you'd expect. This can happen with all frozen foods, and the best way to work around it is to add a bit more herbs and spices.

Chapter 6:

Vegan Sirtfood Recipes

Don't eat animal-based foods? No problem! All of the known Sirtfoods are plant-based, and you'll have no trouble incorporating them into your daily diet. This chapter will feature Sirtfood recipes for vegans, but don't feel limited to these! You can use the recipes from the entire book if you substitute meat, eggs, and dairy with vegan alternatives. Without further ado, here are your Sirtfood meals from breakfast to dinner:

Breakfast

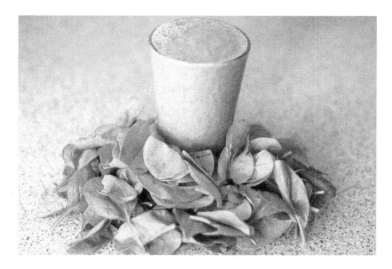

One of the common challenges of crafting a tasty, but calorie-dense breakfast, is to choose foods that are rich in healthy carbs and fiber, but don't have too much fat and sugar. In these recipes, we opted for buckwheat as the main source of carbohydrates, fruits to gain enough fiber, sugar, and vitamins (particularly strawberries), and different nut milks to alter the flavor of the smoothies the way you wish. Aside from adjusting other recipes given in this book, you can choose between these additional options on a vegan diet:

Walnut Chocolate Cupcakes

Ingredients:

- Buckwheat flour, 1 ½ cup
- Sugar, 2 cup
- Cocoa powder, 1 cup
- Salt, ½ tsp
- Almond milk, 1 ½ cup
- Vanilla extract, ½ tsp
- Coconut oil, ½ cup
- Walnuts, 2 tbsp
- Baking powder, 1 tsp

Instructions:

1. Preheat your oven to 180 °C. Lay baking paper on the bottom of a cupcake pan.
2. Mix in flour, cocoa, and sugar and mix through. Mix in the vanilla extract, almond milk, coconut oil, walnuts, and baking powder and mix until the ingredients have combined into an even batter. Add boiling water and beat until it's evenly mixed in with the batter.
3. Your batter should now look quite liquidy, but don't worry!
4. Pour in the batter evenly across cake cases, filling up to ¾ of each case. Bake for up to 18 minutes and let cool.
5. Optionally, you can add vegan icing.

Sirtfood Kale Smoothie

Ingredients:

- Kale, finely chopped, 2 cup
- Raw honey, 2 tsp
- 1 banana
- 1 apple
- Fresh ginger, chopped, 1 tsp
- Half a glass of water, if needed

Instructions:

Blend all the ingredients together and enjoy!

Fruity Matcha Smoothie

Ingredients:

- Matcha powder, 2 tsp
- Milk, 1 ½ cup
- Raw honey, 2 tsp
- Melon, chopped, two cups
- Mint leaves, fresh, 2-3 pieces
- Lemon or lime juice, 1-2 tbsp

Instructions:

Pop all the ingredients into a blender, starting from the liquids to melon, and top with milk, spices, and lemon/lime juice. Blend all together and enjoy!

Fresh SirtFruit Compote

Ingredients:

- Green tea, fresh, ½ cup
- 1 lemon, halved
- 1 chopped apple
- Red grapes, seedless, 1 cup
- Strawberries, 2 cup
- Raw honey, 1 tsp

Instructions:

1. Cook fresh green tea and 1 tsp of raw honey. Add the juice from ½ lemon and let cool.
2. Pour the grapes and strawberries into a bowl and pour the tea over the fruit. Serve after a couple of minutes.

Lunch

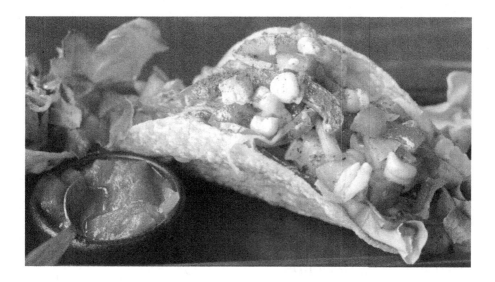

Spicy Sirtfood Ricotta

Ingredients:

- Extra virgin olive oil, 2 tsp
- Unsalted ricotta cheese, 200 g
- Pinch of salt
- Pinch of pepper
- 1 chopped red onion
- 1 tsp of fresh ginger
- 1 finely sliced garlic clove
- 1 finely sliced green chili
- 1 cup diced cherry tomatoes
- ½ tsp ground cumin
- ½ tsp ground coriander
- ½ tsp mild chili powder
- Chopped parsley, ½ cup

- Fresh spinach leaves, 2 cup

Instructions:

1. Heat olive oil in a lidded pan over high heat. Toss in the ricotta cheese, seasoning it with pepper and sea salt. Fry until it turns golden and removes from the pan. Add the onion to the pan and reduce the heat. Fry the onion with chili, ginger, and garlic for around eight minutes and add the chopped tomatoes. Cover with the lid and cook for another five minutes.

2. Add the remaining spices and sea salt to the cheese, put the cheese back into the pan and stir, adding spinach, coriander, and parsley. Cover with the lid and cook for another two minutes.

Sirtfood Baked Potatoes

Ingredients:

- Potatoes, 5 pieces
- Extra virgin olive oil, 2 tbsp
- Organic red wine, 1 tbsp
- 2 finely chopped red onions
- 4 finely chopped garlic cloves
- Finely chopped ginger, 1 tsp
- 1 chopped Bird's eye chili pepper
- Powdered cumin, 1 tbsp
- Ground turmeric, 1 tbsp
- Water, 1 tbsp
- Tomatoes, 2 small cans
- Cocoa powder, 2 tbsp
- Parsley, 2 tbsp
- A pinch of salt

- A pinch of pepper

Instructions:

Start by preheating your oven to 200 °C. Bake potatoes for one hour. In the meantime, fry onions in olive oil for five minutes until they're soft. Add chili, garlic, cumin, and ginger and cook for another minute on low heat. Add a tablespoon of water to prevent dryness. Mix in the tomato, chickpeas, pepper, and cocoa powder and let simmer for 45 minutes until the sauce becomes thick. Add parsley, salt, and pepper and serve with potatoes.

Spicy Quinoa With Kale

Ingredients:
- Canned quinoa, 1 can
- Extra virgin olive oil, 1 tbsp
- 1 sliced red onion
- 3 finely chopped garlic cloves
- 1 finely chopped bird's eye chili
- Turmeric, 2 tsp
- Coconut milk, 2 cup
- Water, 1 cup
- Kale, chopped, 1 cup
- Buckwheat, 2 cup

Instructions:

1. Fry the onions for five minutes in olive oil. Add ginger, garlic, and chili, and fry for another five minutes. Toss in the turmeric and wait for another minute. Then add in the quinoa and coconut milk, pour in a glass of water, and cook for 20 minutes. Add kale and cook for another five minutes.

2. Halfway through cooking the quinoa, fry the buckwheat in water for ten minutes. Drain and serve with the quinoa.

Mediterranean Sirtfood Quinoa

Ingredients:

- Quinoa, 2 cup
- Extra virgin olive oil, 1 tbsp
- Finely chopped garlic cloves, 1 tbsp
- Fresh ginger, chopped, 1 tsp
- 1 sliced bird's eye chili
- 1 sliced red bell pepper
- Ground turmeric, ½ tsp
- Ground cumin, 1 tsp
- A pinch of salt
- A pinch of pepper
- Chopped kale, 1 cup
- Lemon juice, 2 tbsp

Instructions:

Start off by cooking the quinoa. Pour into a pot, cover with two parts water, and bring to a boil. Let it boil for up to thirty minutes. During the last five minutes, pan-fry the vegetables except kale in olive oil for up to five minutes. Once the vegetables have softened, add cumin, paprika, turmeric, salt, and pepper. Stir through and insert quinoa. Stir again, add vegetable stock, and pan-fry until the excess liquid vapors out. Serve and enjoy!

Eggplant and Potatoes in Red Wine

Ingredients:

- 1 large diced potato
- Finely chopped parsley, 2 tsp
- 1 sliced red onion
- Sliced kale, 1 cup
- 1 finely chopped garlic clove
- Sliced eggplant, 2 cup
- Vegetable stock, 1 ½ cup
- Tomato sauce, 1 tsp
- Extra virgin olive oil, 1 tbsp

Instructions:

1. Preheat your oven to 220 °C.
2. Boil the potatoes for five minutes, drain, and roast in the oven for 45 minutes on 1 tsp of extra virgin olive oil. Turn potatoes over every ten minutes so that they cook evenly. Add chopped parsley once the potatoes are done.
3. Stir-fry the garlic, onions, and eggplant on olive oil for up to five minutes. Add the vegetable stock and tomato sauce, bring to a boil, and let simmer up to 15 minutes on low medium heat.
4. Serve with potatoes.

Dinner

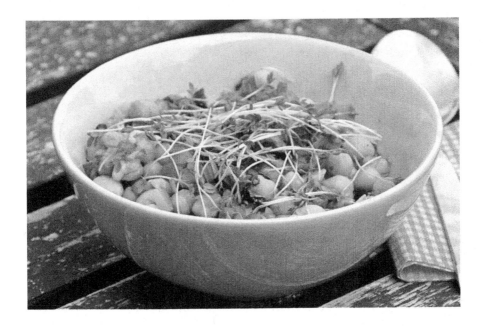

Potatoes With Onion Rings in Red Wine

Ingredients:

- Diced potatoes, 3 cup
- Extra virgin olive oil, 1 tbsp
- Finely chopped parsley, ½ tbsp
- Red wine, 1 tbsp
- Vegetable stock, 150ml
- Tomato sauce, 1 tsp
- 1 sliced red onion
- Kale, sliced, 1 cup
- A pinch of salt
- A pinch of pepper
- 1 chopped bird's eye chili

Instructions:

1. Boil the potatoes for up to five minutes and drain. Roast at 22o °C for 45 minutes. Add the parsley after taking the potatoes out of the oven.

2. Fry the onions for up to seven minutes in 1 tsp of olive oil and add kale and garlic. Add vegetable stock and let boil for up to two minutes. Serve alongside potatoes.

Sweet Potatoes With Grilled Tofu and Mushrooms

Ingredients:

- Tofu, 14 oz
- Chicken stock, 1 cup
- Buckwheat flour, 1 tbsp
- Water, 1 tbsp
- Red wine, 1 tbsp
- Brown sugar, 1 tsp
- Tomato sauce, 1 tbsp
- Soy sauce, 1 tbsp
- 1 finely chopped garlic clove
- Ginger, finely chopped, 1 tsp
- Extra virgin olive oil, 1 tbsp
- Mushrooms, sliced, 1 cup
- 1 sliced red onion
- Kale, chopped, 2 cup
- Sweet potato, diced, 400 g
- Buckwheat, 1 cup
- Chopped parsley, 2 tbsp
- Vegetable stock, 2 cup

Instructions:

1. Drain tofu by wrapping it in kitchen paper as you prepare other ingredients.
2. Cook buckwheat in vegetable stock. Add red wine, the tomato sauce, soy sauce, brown sugar, ginger, and garlic.
3. Stir-fry mushrooms for up to three minutes until cooked through. Add tofu and stir fry until the cheese turns golden. Remove from the pan and set aside.
4. Add the onions and stir fry for two minutes, upon which you'll add the diced sweet potatoes. Add more water or vegetable stock if needed, and add the sauce a minute or two before finishing. Combine the remaining ingredients and serve.

Buckwheat Stew

Ingredients:

- 1 finely chopped red onion
- 1 finely chopped large carrot
- 1 finely chopped garlic clove
- Finely chopped celery, 3 tbsp
- Extra virgin olive oil, 1 tbsp
- 1 finely chopped garlic clove
- 1 finely chopped bird's eye chili
- Vegetable stock, 2 cups
- Rosemary, ½ tsp
- Basil, ½ tsp
- Dill, ½ tsp
- Celery, finely chopped, 1 tbsp
- Canned tomatoes, 400 g
- Buckwheat, 2 cup
- Kale, chopped, ½ cup

- Parsley, chopped, 1 tbsp

Instructions:

1. Fry the onions, garlic, chili, celery, carrot, and spice herbs in olive oil on low heat. Once the onion turns soft, add the vegetable stock and tomato sauce. Once the stock boils, add the buckwheat and let simmer for another half an hour. Add kale and parsley during the last five minutes.

Cooking vegan on a Sirtfood regimen may look challenging at first, but the process can become easier and fun with some creativity. As with all other recipes, you're welcome to switch, substitute, and adjust ingredients per your own taste. Here are a couple of extra tips for more cooking inspiration:

- **Go for avocados.** Avocados are very popular for those on a vegan diet because they supply plenty of natural fats and replenishing vitamins. But, for some, they're expensive or unavailable to buy on a regular basis. If this is your case, you can use bananas, melons, or sweet potatoes instead (depending on the recipe).
- **Add nut butters.** If some of the recipes given in this chapter are too lean for your taste, you can add nut butters or crushed nuts to the recipes. This will increase their flavor and add extra fat.
- **Cook vegetables carefully.** It might be tempting to let a dish simmer a couple minutes longer, but it's always better to steam or stir-fry as short as possible. Your vegetables are ready as soon as you can run a fork through them, and there's no reason to cook a second longer.
- **Shuffle milks.** You may get tired of coconut and almond milk. If you do, it's perfectly fine to use substitutes. Oat milk is one of the options you can go for as it won't significantly alter the

flavor of the dish, but it will add sweetness. You can use soy milk as well, as it has a more neutral flavor.

- **Explore mushrooms**. Mushrooms are a great, lean source of protein, and you can choose from a long list of different species. They are easy and quick to prepare, and taste great overall. However, make sure to get mushrooms only from reliable brands and suppliers. They carry a risk from poisoning if grown near inedible mushrooms, and can cause great stomach discomfort past their expiry date. They are also heavily reliant on soil quality, which is why you should only buy organic ones. If you don't like mushrooms, you can always substitute them for artichokes.

- **Spice it up!** The recipes in this chapter feature a limited number of spices to ensure neutral flavors that will suit the majority of tastes. However, you can add any and all spices you like.

- **Improvise with flaxseed.** If you want to substitute animal-based ingredients from this cookbook, you can do so by mixing water and flaxseed meals in 3:1 ratio. This substitute will be great to substitute eggs so you can make your own vegan omelets and pancakes.

- **Invest in organic foods.** The Sirtfood program doesn't last forever, and since you'll be on a limited 1,000-1,500 calorie regimen, you won't use large quantities of foods, oils, and spices. Organic extra virgin olive oil, as expensive as it can get, is a great choice. You'll use it in almost all of your meals, and it's rich in nutrients and healthy fats. The same goes for coconut oil and herbs. Organic produce, while being more costly, is also richer in taste and smell, and it will secure a flavorful meal.

Now, the best is saved for the very end. The list of available vegan Sirtfood meals doesn't end with this chapter. In this chapter, you learned what to eat for breakfast, lunch, and dinner. But, what about those moments when you start craving sugar and sweets? This book's got you covered! In the last chapter of this book, you'll find recipes for delicious sweets and pancakes.

Chapter 7:

Sirtfood Desserts

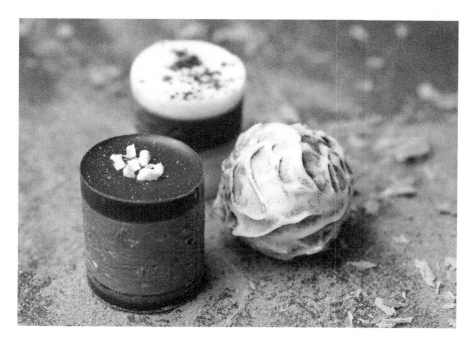

It's one thing to eat clean and lean, but a completely different story to completely deprive yourself of sweets. The majority of diet plans fail because they don't acknowledge cravings for sweets. On most occasions, these cravings can be soothed by snacking on fruits, but not always. At times, you'll want to eat a delicious chocolate cake, or have some saucy pancakes. In this chapter, you'll find a couple of dessert recipes that are all based on Sirtfoods. These recipes are low-calorie, healthy, and easy to make. Enjoy!

Sirtfood Walnut Balls

Ingredients:

- Cocoa or almond milk, 1-2 tbsp
- Medjool dates, 2 cup
- Walnuts, 2 cup
- Vanilla, either one pod or 1 tsp extract
- Dark chocolate or cocoa nibs, 1 ½ cup
- Extra Virgin Olive Oil, 1 tbsp
- Turmeric, 1 tbsp
- Cocoa Powder, 1 tbsp

Instructions:

Pop the chocolate and walnuts into your blender and process into a fine powder, adding milk and the remaining ingredients. Feel free to add more milk if the consistency of the mixture feels too thick, because this may depend on the freshness of the ingredients and individual package characteristics. Form the mixture into balls or any other shape and size of your choosing and roll in desiccated coconut and/or cocoa. This dessert can last up for a week in your fridge.

Sirtfood Brownies

This delicious treat will take only five minutes to make! You will need to mix in a shortlist of ingredients.

Ingredients:

- Walnuts, whole, 2 cup
- Almond milk, ½ tbsp
- Rum, 2 tsp

- Almonds, 1 cup
- Medjool dates, 2 ½ cup
- Vanilla extract, 1 tsp
- A pinch of sea salt
- Cacao powder, 1 cup

Instructions:

Pour all ingredients together into a blender and blend until combined. Shape into balls, and either keep in your fridge for about two hours or keep in your freezer for around 30 minutes.

Sirtfood Chocolate Mousse

Ingredients:

- Dark chocolate, 85%, 250 g
- 6 eggs
- Black coffee, strong, 4 tbsp
- Almond milk, 4 tbsp
- Chocolate flakes

Instructions:

Place a bowl over a pan of simmering water. Melt the chocolate inside it, while paying attention not to touch the water with the bottom of the bowl. Remove the bowl and allow the chocolate to cool. Once the chocolate has cooled off, add egg yolks and the coffee and almond milk. Whisk with a mixer and add the egg whites gradually, while slowly mixing it with a spoon. Pour the mousse into glasses, flatten the surface, cover with thin foil, and cool for two hours. The mouse can also stay overnight. Sprinkle with chocolate flakes before serving.

Chocolate Sauce and Strawberry Pancakes

Ingredients:

Batter

- 1 egg
- Milk, 350 ml
- Buckwheat flour, 5 oz
- Extra virgin olive oil, 1 tbsp
- Dark chocolate, 85%, 3.5 oz

Sauce

- Milk for chocolate sauce, 85 ml
- Double cream, 1 tbsp
- Extra virgin olive oil for the sauce, 1 tbsp
- Chopped walnuts, 1 cup
- Chopped strawberries, 4 cup

Instructions:

1. Start by making the pancake batter. Mix in all the ingredients for the batter, pour into a blender and blend until smooth. You should have a batter of medium thickness, not too runny.
2. Start making the sauce. Place a bowl over a pan of simmering water, while making sure that the bottom of the bowl doesn't touch the water. Place the chocolate in the bowl and melt over the steam. Once the chocolate has melted, add the milk and whisk for a minute. Add the olive oil and double cream.
3. Start making pancakes. Heat a frying pan until it starts to smoke. Insert extra virgin olive oil, and pour some batter into the center. Spread the batter across the surface of the pan. Cook for one minute on each side. Once the pancakes start

lifting along the edges of the pan, use a spatula to lift and flip to the other side.

4. Once the pancakes are ready, spread the strawberries as you wish and roll the pancake. Layer the desired amount of sauce on top.

Cocoa and Medjool Dates Snacks

If you're one of those people who enjoy your afternoon sweets, these bite-sized cocoa balls will be a perfect substitute for your usual sweets.

Ingredients:

- Dark chocolate, 70-85%, ½ cup
- Walnuts, 1 cup
- Pitted Medjool dates, 1 ½ cups
- Cocoa powder, 1 tbsp
- Vanilla extract, 1 tsp
- Water, 2 tbsp
- Extra virgin olive oil, 1 tbsp

Instructions:

Pop all the ingredients into a blender and blend until you get a homogenous, ball-shaped batter. Roll individual balls by pulling out bits from the batter and refrigerate for at least an hour before serving. Optionally, you can roll the balls in coconut or cocoa powder.

Congratulations! You've reached the end of your Sirtfood journey! Hopefully, the final chapters of this book gave you enough guidance and options to enjoy each and every of your meals.

Conclusion

Congratulations! You now know how to follow the Sirtfood diet diligently and lose weight healthily and consistently. The main purpose of this book was to show you the basics of this diet concept, remove doubts, and give instructions for how to apply the techniques so that you burn fat and feel great throughout the process.

First, you learned where the Sirtfood diet originated, and where its true significance lies. You discovered that weight loss is much more than a "calories in, calories out" equation. Through this book, you now realize that the main reasons why you have trouble losing weight lie in more than just the foods you eat. You learned that, oftentimes, the inability to invest time, effort, and resources into diet planning, and trying to follow through with a complicated diet regiment leads to failure. Now you know that your diet needs to be well-balanced, nutrient-dense, tasty, and easy to follow so that you spark your metabolism and enjoy your foods. Most importantly, you can now recognize that an unhealthy diet, despite being restrictive, won't lead to permanent weight loss. You learned that calorie restriction slows down metabolism if and when macronutrients like carbohydrates, fats, and protein are reduced to a minimum.

You read about how losing weight doesn't necessarily mean losing fat, and you can be both lean and obese at the same time, as calorie deprivation leads to the loss of your muscle mass. And that's where the Sirtfood diet kicks in.

In the first chapter of this book, you learned that the Sirtfood diet is designed to create all the necessary conditions for activating your "skinny gene," or SIRT 1 gene. We explored how this gene links to cellular health, longevity, and metabolism. A very fine set of circumstances needs to be created for this gene to be activated, and this process starts with the intake of sirtuin-boosting foods. You are now aware that certain foods contain important compounds, such as sirtuin-activating resveratrol, that directly link to fat-burning. More importantly, you can now see that this beneficial substance enables you to exercise more while eating less, shift to burning fat instead of burning muscles for fuel, and lose weight healthily in this way. Remember, the main reasons why popular fat diets fail aren't because you're not good at dieting, but because they're poorly designed. They drive your body into starvation and temporarily deplete water supplies, which are then quickly replenished, leading to the infamous yo-yo effect.

But, as you read, there is one way to prevent this and make weight loss quickly visible, consistent, and permanent. The right way is to hack fat burning. As you learned, this is one of the most difficult things to do. After all, our bodies love storing fat, just as we like storing food in the freezer. Making your body let go of these supplies is difficult.

After reading, you now recognize that this is possible if you carefully measure and provide the finely-balanced circumstances and influences to lose weight. First, you learned, you need a calorie deficit to alert your metabolism. Then, you need to supply restricted and limited amounts of evenly distributed macronutrients for your body not to go in 'starvation' mode and shut down metabolism, but instead, just reach for burning more glucose and fat. Then, as you learned, activity and exercises are needed to push the metabolic processes over the edge, and finely trigger fat burning. But, there is still a missing element. How does one exercise more and eat less? just eating less is difficult enough, let alone being hungry and exercising.

Not anymore! The answer to this enigma is given in this no-nonsense, comprehensive diet plan. Simply, eat a lot of foods that boost sirtuin and contain resveratrol. These compounds, when introduced into a body that's, quite literally, "stretched too thin" with borderline calorie restriction and moderate exercise, actually flip the switch between your body burning glucose to fat burning. All that, with the simple use of common foods, that are quite available and affordable in your nearest grocery store.

With this knowledge, the time came for you to learn how to apply this diet. You learned that, according to some, the Sirtfood diet consists of two phases, followed by optional maintenance, or three phases, in which the third is called "Sirtfood for life."

During the first phase of the diet, you're allowed a single meal and three servings of the Sirtfood Green Juice. That probably wasn't pleasant to acknowledge. But, the more you read about the phase, the more it became clear that, while lean, this stage of the diet is also delicious and satisfying, particularly if you balance your foods well. Remember, with 90 calories being in a single green juice, meaning 270 calories deducted at the start, you'll have to make your meal quite a large one. It will consist of 730 calories, 365 of it being carbs, 180 protein, and 180 fat. Now, that's one tasty meal! Perhaps, with this insight, it became clear that, while you may be on a restricted diet, your body most certainly doesn't have to be nutrient-deprived. Still, the first week of the diet is intense for the majority, which is why it's recommended to exercise lightly and choose walking in the fresh air instead of vigorous cardio exercising.

Once your body gets used to a calorie deficit, you will start the second phase of the diet. During this phase, as you know, you will eat 1,500 calories, evenly distributed across three meals. Two snacks are allowed, with your choices being dark chocolate, strawberries, Medjool dates, celery, and many other delicious options. A glass of wine of course, before bedtime, also recommended to not only help you fall asleep but also help burn fat.

As you learned, during the second phase of the diet, you should have two Sirtfood Green juices (180 calories), and the rest of the calories distributed to 440 calorie meals, with a 50:25:25 macronutrient ratio. Remember, the more Sirt foods that are introduced in your daily meal plan, the more you lose weight over time.

There are a total of 20 sirtuin-boosting foods, although you don't have to eat all of them in a single day. You learned that, while your meals should mainly consist of these foods, you can also eat meat, dairy, eggs, and other fruits, vegetables, beans, and legumes you like. Then, the time came for you to figure out how to cook Sirtfoods. This book presented you with a menu and recipes for carnivore, vegan, and vegetarian, and also gave you a couple of dessert recipes so that you stay full and feel satisfied throughout the second phase.

If you tried making any of these recipes, you probably noticed that balanced cooking is easier than it first seemed. Over time, you'll know how many cups and tablespoons of each make for a balanced Sirtfood meal, and you'll also learn to adjust these foods to your taste. In this book, you also found some suggestions for alternatives, in case you don't like or don't have certain ingredients in your kitchen.

The final, and perhaps the most interesting topic we've covered, is long-term weight maintenance. You learned that many psychological factors are affecting your eating habits. Perhaps, you have been brought up to cook spicy and gourmet, using more fat and overall larger quantities than needed. Maybe, you were raised to think that a house isn't a home without a warm ambiance, and a kitchen overflowing with delicious meals. Maybe, you have been trained to think that not having a kitchen full of food means a cold, empty, or a poor home. Maybe, you like a welcoming atmosphere, and one of the ways to create is to cook and bake regularly, even when there is no guest to greet. As you now know, all of these influences may have caused you to eat much more than you need. You may feel compelled to cook all the time, and since the food is there, why not eat?

Or, perhaps, your life is too stressful, you are anxious and you feel like your fear, anger, or sadness are overwhelming, so you eat to calm down? Maybe you simply haven't learned other ways to reward yourself or celebrate, so you eat whenever you feel good? Whichever the reason, you learned that eating out of habit, unconsciously, or to cope, links not only with weight gain but also with poor mental health and productivity. You now see that emotional and habitual eating may cause you to eat without even noticing it, or to lose touch with your biological appetite, and eat quickly on auto-pilot.

Now that you're aware of all of these influences, the question is, how to stop them from coming back once you're done with the program?

The answer is by becoming mindful of your eating, learning healthier strategies to cope with feelings, and focusing on your eating intuition, all framed in the healthy balance among macronutrients. The first weeks of the diet will help you focus on your biological appetite, break your sugar addiction, and start finding pleasure in natural sugars to soothe your cravings. With a neat eating schedule and a regular full stomach, you'll be less tempted to eat spontaneously. Once you're done with the program, you will have long learned how to cook healthily, how to shop nutritiously, and how to adjust and plan meals to account for good and bad days. This will make it much easier to stay committed to eating balanced and inserting Sirtfoods wherever and whenever you can. Long-term weight loss will still demand a caloric deficit, which is why increasing your daily calorie intake should be done patiently and gradually. Ideally, you'll add 100-200 more calories to your daily menu per week, until you reach your daily limit. This book also provided you with a formula to calculate your daily calorie needs, which you can use to monitor your calorie intake and decide how big of a deficit you want to make. As long as there are at least 200 calories more spent than eaten, you will contribute to losing weight healthily.

Hopefully, this book helped you gain a deeper understanding not only of the Sirtfood diet but also of proper eating and cooking overall. Finally, this book included some general tips for healthy cooking, so that you preserve the majority of the sirtuin-boosting nutrients in your plants. You learned that you shouldn't expose your veggies to extreme heat and that you should opt for microwaving whenever you can so that you don't lose the water-soluble nutrients.

You also discovered an easy way to control your portion sizes, and that is to purchase appropriately sized bowls and plates to match your calorie intake for each of the food groups. While this will make it easier to control how much you eat, you also learned that there is an easy way to balance the different components, too. Simply, put veggies on one half of your plate, including starchy ones, and then have protein and fats take up the remaining two-quarters of your plate. When eating out, as you learned, you can start by ordering half of a portion, eating slowly, and adding more if you decide that there's a need.

There's so much to account for if you want to lose weight healthily! It's not easy, I admit it. I want to leave you with a final note of support. I would like you to be patient and kind to yourself throughout this process. Remember, the reasons why you may have become obese or unhealthy in the first were probably outside of your awareness. So please, never believe anyone who tells you that you are lazy for not losing weight, or that you overeat because you don't care for your health. The majority of reasons why you might be overweight are out of your control, but the weight loss isn't. While you're not to blame for being overweight, and that certainly doesn't speak about your personality, you are the only person who can make a change.

Devote to learning about proper eating, and making unconscious choices conscious ones. Track your thoughts, moods, and meals, to find a connection and prevent yourself from slipping back into old habits. More importantly, nurture your digestive health to regain that healthy connection with your eating intuition, or gut-brain axis, as scientists like to call it. Do this by introducing as many plants and probiotics as possible into your diet enabling your gut to better communicate with your mind to create sensations of hunger, satiety, and pleasure when you truly need it, and in the form of healthy cravings for fruits, lean meat, and vegetables.

Use all that you have learned and read in these pages to take back control of your life and your diet. You possess all the knowledge you need; the choice is yours!

References

Chalkiadaki, A., Igarashi, M., Nasamu, A. S., Knezevic, J., & Guarente, L. (2014). Muscle-specific SIRT1 gain-of-function increases slow-twitch fibers and ameliorates pathophysiology in a mouse model of duchenne muscular dystrophy. *PLoS Genet*, 10(7), e1004490.

Horwath, C., Hagmann, D., & Hartmann, C. (2019). Intuitive eating and food intake in men and women: Results from the Swiss food panel study. *Appetite*, 135, 61-71.

Goggins, A., & Matten, G. (2017). *The Sirtfood Diet*. Simon and Schuster.

Kuningas, M., Putters, M., Westendorp, R. G., Slagboom, P. E., & Van Heemst, D. (2007). SIRT1 gene, age-related diseases, and mortality: the Leiden 85-plus study. *The Journals of Gerontology Series A: Biological Sciences and Medical Sciences*, 62(9), 960-965.

Lagouge, M., Argmann, C., Gerhart-Hines, Z., Meziane, H., Lerin, C., Daussin, F., ... & Geny, B. (2006). Resveratrol improves mitochondrial function and protects against metabolic disease by activating SIRT1 and PGC-1α. *Cell*, 127(6), 1109-1122.

Maier, A., Vickers, Z., & Inman, J. J. (2007). Sensory-specific satiety, its crossovers, and subsequent choice of potato chip flavors. *Appetite*, 49(2), 419-428.

McClung, C. A. (2013). How might circadian rhythms control mood? Let me count the ways... *Biological psychiatry*, 74(4), 242-249.

Niccolai, E., Boem, F., Russo, E., & Amedei, A. (2019). The Gut–Brain Axis in the Neuropsychological Disease Model of Obesity: A

Classical Movie Revised by the Emerging Director "Microbiome". *Nutrients*, 11(1), 156.

Stefanick, M. L. (1993). Exercise and weight control. *Exercise and Sport Sciences Reviews*, 21, 363-396.

Waller, G., & Matoba, M. (1999). Emotional eating and eating psychopathology in nonclinical groups: A cross-cultural comparison of women in Japan and the United Kingdom. *International Journal of Eating Disorders*, 26(3), 333-340.